KILLING CANCER –
NOT PEOPLE

KILLING CANCER – NOT PEOPLE

WHAT I WOULD DO
IF I HAD CANCER

ROBERT G. WRIGHT

DIRECTOR
AMERICAN ANTI-CANCER INSTITUTE

Forewords by
Bill Henderson, Lynn Jennings and Chris Young

Second Edition

Copyright © 2011 by Robert G. Wright

Notice of Rights

Printed and bound in the United States of America

ISBN 978-0-578-06184-9

CONTENTS

WHAT OTHERS
ARE SAYING ABOUT
"KILLING CANCER – NOT PEOPLE"

"This book is an amazing source of information for anyone researching the definitive relationship that nutrition bears upon our health. The link between alkalinity and cellular oxygen was clearly defined and the frequent question, 'what should I do and what should I stop doing,' was clearly addressed. The author, Bob Wright, explains several potent natural cancer treatments. He talks about the importance of vitamin D and even goes into details about the Navarro Urine Test, which is a great natural and non-invasive method to test for cancer.

"The book is well organized and contains *TRUTH*, despite the fact that it contains information that is not widely known and could be considered 'outside the box.' Having written a book on cancer treatments myself, I was impressed with Mr. Wright's thoroughness and clarity. I honestly believe that whether or not you have cancer, this book is a must have!"

Ty Bollinger, Author
"Cancer – Step Outside the Box"

"Thank you, Robert Wright, for including in this courageous book you have written information on how your readers can treat cancer practically and inexpensively using the Brazilian Aloe

Aborescens Immune Recipe I publicized in two books. I have seen it cure cancer of all parts of the body for patients on five different continents. My files are filled with letters from users from all over the world testifying of their curing cancer. The therapeutic medicinal properties in this aloe species rebuild the immune system and gently detoxify the body of impurities so the body heals itself through nutrition. It is evidenced-based, natural medicine published in official scientific publications."

Father Romano Zago, OFM (Order of Friars Minor),
Brazilian scholar and author of the book, "Cancer Can Be Cured"

"The minute I read the first page of Bob Wright's book '*Killing Cancer – Not People*,' I immediately knew I had struck oil. His book is a true testament to an effective alternative cancer treatment. Two of the factors that make this book such a page-turner are the meticulous knowledge and facts the writer has accumulated throughout his decades of research. Each argument against the three types of traditional cancer treatments is heavily saturated with facts – testifying to the wrongs of traditional cancer treatment. '*Killing Cancer – Not People*' is a pure dose of truth and is a must for anyone who desires a healthy body, mind and spirit."

John Foote, Pacific Lutheran University

"Being involved in health and wellness as CNC's, we are continually reading and studying literature on the subject. However, from page 1 of Robert Wright's, '*Killing Cancer – Not People*,' we were absolutely hooked and fascinated. His straight-forward, no B.S. style, allows readers to fully understand every point in the book. And we love the way you can connect with the author – to where you almost feel as if you are in a one-on-one conversation between him and you. And all the while he speaks the truth without hesitation. This book – and the message in it – is exactly what America, and the world, needs. He exposes the truth behind the lies and dangers of 'conventional treatments,' while giving the readers alternative choices that, in his decades of research, have been proven to work.

"This book is an absolute must-read for everyone – cancer or not! Too many lives have been lost due to being misinformed and lied to. The way it is written really drives these shocking truths home, even if you already know them to be true. He absolutely has a gift to be shared with the world, and this book WILL be life-changing and mind-altering across the globe. Our passion for health, wellness, and truth has been re-ignited after reading this book. Thank you, Robert, for this incredible gift of truth!"

Joshua and Anna Scurry, CNC's, reverseage.org

"In his book entitled, '*Killing Cancer – Not People,*' Robert Wright spills out – in a simple way from A to Z – the many different ways of healing cancer in a natural way. He gives you information on how you can take small actions every day to heal yourself of cancer – as well as to prevent cancer. It is a 'must read' for everybody."

Lea Yekutiel, Author, "Making the Breast of It"

"I talk to people with cancer every day. At our pharmacy, we strive to inform and educate our clients regarding alternative cancer treatments and supplements. Most people don't know what to do or where to start. I suggest, '*Killing Cancer – Not People,*' as the best place to start. The book is easily understood and gets to the point with the truth about cancer and how to heal it. I consider it my cancer Bible. My copy is tagged so I can go right to a certain topic and read to our clients. I use the book in our Tuesday health lectures and our Wednesday night water lectures. This book is exactly what I needed to help spread the word that there are natural ways to heal cancer."

Barbara Hubbard, Town Center Compounding Pharmacy

"'*Killing Cancer – Not People,*' is a must read for everyone! This book provides insightful information that educates and empowers everyone in the fight against cancer. Bob Wright's vision to present the 'truth' is very detailed. I highly recommend this book to anyone, not just those diagnosed with cancer."

Dave Zuro, Crestwood, Illinois

"THANK YOU so much for writing your book, '*Killing Cancer – Not People.*' This book is incredible, life-changing, with heart-felt wisdom – and so encouraging, giving everyone HOPE!!! The same hope, back in the Garden of Eden, that God gave us with fresh fruits and vegetables, clean air, the right type of water, exercise, and no stress. God intended Adam and Eve to live forever, without the doctor and drugs! Your book sets the stage for that abundant life on earth. We share your book with so many people. The results have changed my life. And you are right – I couldn't put the book down. Thanks, again. May God continue to bless you and others with your book."

Mark Thomas

"Bob Wright's book gave me so much hope and was very empowering! What a fantastic resource for those of us who have had the 'C' word pronounced over us. It's a road map for alternative treatment that I will share with anyone who is in need. Thank you – what a blessing!"

Karen Ellis, Regional VP, Arbonne International

"This pharmacy is truly a clinical setting with pharmacists available to talk to patients. One of the most important things we do in our practice is triage information for many people. The people we see want to be more proactive in their health care. Therefore, what a wonderful resource this book is for people who are on the journey to take control and responsibility for their cancer. '*Killing Cancer – Not People,*' is the first book we recommend to our patients who are seeking information. The websites are particularly helpful. Eight years ago we lost our daughter to Hodgkin's Lymphoma. I know one of the biggest issues for people is what to do, when to do it, and can I trust it. In addition, I realized we were not capable of clear thinking while we were in the process of her cancer treatment. In my opinion, we should all have the right in this country to freedom of choice in our medical care – and not to be laughed at and ridiculed for our choices. I pray God's Blessing on anyone who makes the courageous choice to take responsibility for their care."

Ronald E. Partain, RPH, C.C.N, Compounding Pharmacist,
Certified Clinical Nutritionist, Town Center
Compounding Pharmacy

DISCLAIMER

PLEASE ascribe to the following before reading the contents of this book:

It is a shame that in this day and age we have to apologize for and, essentially, "disavow" what we believe are the truths about cancer and its effective treatments – through disclaimers. The sad fact is that we do – and we must – to placate those that would rather see us in jail than patients who have been healed. With that in mind, please review the following and take it to heart – as much as you can:

I am not a doctor – nor do I play one on T.V. I do not practice medicine, diagnose, treat, or advise sick or diseased patients. Please make no inference through these chapters that I do.

What you will find within the pages of this book is for educational purposes only. There is no intention herein to diagnose, treat or advise you. You should seek these services from qualified and licensed medical professionals and consult with healthcare specialists regarding recommendations in this text.

To the best of my ability, I have utilized experience, real life testimonies, research, and facts and figures that I deem to be true and accurate in the writing of this book. I assume no responsibility if any of the sources or materials herein are not so.

Any statements referencing "alternative" treatments, therapies, protocols or nutritional supplements have not been evaluated by the FDA nor approved by that agency.

There are over 400 known "alternative" treatments for cancer. This book makes no effort to cover each one but, rather, is a compilation of those deemed most important and effective for cancer sufferers. These are what I would use, based upon experience and empirical evidence, if I were diagnosed with cancer. Again, the FDA has not approved these.

No one who has had input regarding this work, be it author, publisher(s), editors, contributors, websites, cancer patients, anti-cancer clinics, or any others, including representatives of the aforementioned, will be liable for damages of any kind that arise out of or in connection with the contents and use of this book. This comprehensive liability limitation is complete and inclusive with respect to any loss or damages that are direct, indirect, or compensatory, and extends to property and claims of third parties.

Please consult your physician prior to beginning any of the treatments, therapies, supplements or protocols mentioned in this book. Utilization of these, or of any of the data and information in this work, implies acceptance of the entirety of this disclaimer.

ACKNOWLEDGEMENTS

VERY few solo human feats, be it the writing of a book or sailing across the ocean, are really accomplished alone. Someone, somewhere, has lent expertise, advice, legwork, emotional support, or hands-on assistance in getting the job done.

This book is no exception. Many hands, ounces of sweat, and a generous portion of tears go into a work such as this, a task that is heartfelt and emotionally charged and, arguably, controversial on several fronts.

No intent is forwarded – nor attempt ever made – within these pages to malign the hard-working American people who are genuinely serving cancer patients through conventional medicine. And many thanks go to those (in anonymity) who have provided their literary expertise, and to others for direction in keeping the message centered, focused, and on course.

To the thousands of board certified medical doctors who have grasped the realization that the efforts of traditional, allopathic medicine are failing our citizens, I offer my sincere appreciation for your move to "the far side" that is wrongly and sadly misnamed "alternative medicine." Unknown to many, naturopaths, chiropractors, herbalists, biological dentists, massage therapists, and a plethora of other natural practitioners, are lending their significant knowledge and understanding to cancer and other human maladies. Their contribution is noted and valued.

Even though it is known and documented that a well-nourished and robust immune system will almost always heal a sick or diseased body, research continues in the laboratories of the world to produce the magic elixir that is the "cure" for cancer. Sadly, through drugs and synthetic intervention, this cure does not – and will never – exist. No, the **real** important advances in research are being done by those who understand that the "secret" lies in what sustains, feeds, and builds up the human frame, and the natural compounds that accomplish this feat. Their work is not recognized by conventional entities and goes unnoticed, unheralded, and, largely, unused. Thank you for your ongoing toil and unappreciated sacrifice that, ultimately, provides man with the answer to cancer.

To my friends at the Independent Cancer Research Foundation, in particular, Mike Vrentas, Bill Henderson, and Webster Kehr (the Cancer Tutor), your expertise and continued endurance is much appreciated and often undervalued.

Dr. Eduardo De la Maria, Ph.D., your input and vast knowledge regarding the cause and effective treatment of cancer have been of great value and will prove their worthiness to all in the cancer industry – and the American People – over time.

To the Board, employees, volunteers, and "servants" of the American Anti-Cancer Institute, thank you for your continuous labor in bringing the truth about cancer, its prevention and healing protocols, to the forefront of the mistitled "war on cancer."

My special thanks to Mike Adams, the legendary "Health Ranger," who, with the dedicated workers at *NaturalNews.com*, continues to invest himself in the tireless work that, ultimately, results in the truth being revealed. Mike, his staff, and those like them, are the true heroes of "fact finding" and "revelation" as it pertains to health care/sick care in our country (especially cancer), and their unceasing aggression toward what is wrong in America is, indeed, critical and refreshing. Mike is the author of *"Welcome to the Town of Allopath."*

There are many others who have participated in some way to bring this work to cancer sufferers throughout the United States – and the world. You know who you are and my gratitude is deep and sincere. Thank you for your support and acknowledgement of the words herein.

And, lastly, to my wife, Linda, my continued love and appreciation for putting up with me and my "controlled rage" against an establishment that has produced significant pain and suffering in our combined families and those of so many other Americans across this great land. I don't know how you do it.

IN MEMORIAM

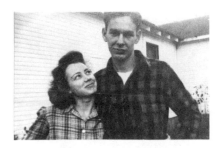

**In memory of my parents,
Marilyn Wright Flaherty and Eugene Wright.**

THANK you, Mom, for the unconditional love you bestowed upon me no matter how near or far. Thank you, Dad, for teaching us what it means to be brave. It is those gifts of love and courage that have inspired me to do the research and pursue the truth of a better way to heal ourselves of cancer and other diseases. If my efforts serve, even in some small way, to enlighten and heal my fellow man, I say, "that's just peachy."

FOREWORD

"KILLING CANCER – NOT PEOPLE"

IN my 12 years of helping cancer patients heal themselves, I become more convinced every day that there is only one reason people die of cancer. It is lack of information. With books like the one you hold in your hand, there is now no excuse for that. Here Bob Wright has given you everything you need to know about cancer – what causes it, how to heal it, how to avoid it, how corrupt the medical and pharmaceutical industries are – everything.

I've seen many friends and relatives, including my former wife and my youngest son, die needlessly because of the "sick care" ignorance of well-meaning doctors. There is no more important message to learn and teach your loved ones than "...only you can heal yourself." This book will give you all the ammunition you need to inform them and yourself. They still may not listen, but at least you will have done your best to give them the resources they need.

Bob gives you here a fabulous "User's Manual" for your body. He says he's giving you "the truth" and he's right. I've read dozens of books on healing cancer using natural substances – the why and how. This is the best. I've written and published three such books myself. This is the best. *Bar none.*

Don't miss the vision Bob has for the mission of his American Anti-Cancer Institute, University and Immune Clinic (Chapter 13). What a great blessing it will be for cancer patients to have a wonderful resource like that to rely on! I only hope I live long enough to see it born and thriving.

We have to make what we now call "alternative medicine" the primary healing choice for all of us. It is our only hope to recover our health and our nation's economic health. Enjoy this book and apply Bob's guidance. You will be very glad you found it.

Bill Henderson
Author, *Cure Your Cancer, Cancer-Free* and *How To Heal Almost Any Cancer At Home For $5.15 A Day*

http://www.Beating-Cancer-Gently.com

FOREWORD TWO

"KILLING CANCER – NOT PEOPLE"

"Two roads diverged in a wood and I – I took the one less traveled by. And that has made all the difference."

Robert Frost

I met the author of this book, Bob Wright, at the 2010 Cancer Control Society Convention. A few weeks before the convention I received an email copy of the first edition of his book, *Killing Cancer – Not People*. Once I opened the book, I could not put it down. This book is not just for people with cancer. It is also for doctors, nurses and other healthcare providers who are looking for alternatives for their patients. It is the book I wish I could have written.

I am a board-certified, family practice physician with an alternative practice in Texas. I am also the medical consultant for Camelot Cancer Care in Tulsa, Oklahoma. I am taking the road less traveled. When Bob asked if I would be willing to write an introduction for the second edition, I wondered what I could say. Bob suggested I write about myself. You can thank me now. I considered, I wrote, I deleted. This book is not about me; it is about beating cancer.

Almost everyone has had a family member or friend with cancer. Several years ago my mother was diagnosed with lung cancer. My mother is an intelligent woman but she is from a generation that still believes traditional medicine has all the answers. Surgery was not an option. Her oncologists recommended she receive chemotherapy and radiation treatments.

I passionately argued against the recommended prophylactic radiation to her brain, which, thankfully, she did not do. After receiving the prescribed regimen of chemotherapy and radiation (not to her brain), her post treatment CT scans showed residual tumor in her lung. I convinced her to begin some alternative therapy. I am happy to say that all of her follow-up studies show no residual or recurrent tumor. Why did my mother opt for traditional therapy? I believe she was scared for her life and I know she was not offered any alternative options by her "trusted doctors."

The cancer industry angers me. I hear this again and again. When a patient is diagnosed with cancer, they feel forced into making immediate decisions on treatment. They are intimidated into thinking that a delay to make a decision will be the cause for failure of the prescribed treatment. Cancer doesn't occur "overnight." It is generally accepted that cancer has been present for many years before symptoms or signs develop. A short delay to explore your options is not going to be the cause of a failure of chemotherapy or radiation to affect a cure.

I object to the way that patients are frightened into believing that the only chance they have is with one of the "golden three." Worse, is the fact that patients are not told that there are alternatives. The gold standards for traditional cancer treatment in the United States are surgery, chemotherapy and radiation. In other words, slash, poison, and burn. When I say "standard," what I mean to say is "sanctioned." The only "gold" about these treatments is the cost. The American Cancer Society (ACS) projected that there would be 1,529,560 new cases of cancer in 2010. When you consider the cost of traditional treatment, it's obvious that cancer is big business.

If surgery, chemo and radiation were effective treatment options; if there was value to be had in the form of extension and quality of life; then certainly it would be worth the price. It is my opinion that, of the golden three, only surgery seems to be helpful (in early stage cancer). In December, 2004, *Clinical Oncology* published a study which reviewed the data of adult patients receiving chemotherapy for cancer in the United States and Australia (in 1998). The five-year survival rate for adult cancer patients receiving chemotherapy was found to be 2.3% (Australia) and 2.1% (United States). These are disappointing results. In 2010, the American Cancer Society predicted that there would be 569,490 deaths due to cancer in the United States.

In the event that you were one of the 2.1% that survived the first 5 years, what will keep you from having a recurrent or new cancer? A functioning, intact immune system is the only way to prevent recurrent or new cancer. Chemotherapy and radiation treatments increase your risk of developing a new cancer by suppressing or destroying your immune system. Of the alternative therapies discussed in this book, none will have an adverse effect on your immune system.

I believe that the best treatment for cancer is prevention. This book is an excellent resource for anyone who is interested in preventing or treating cancer alternatively. The decision to go traditional, alternative, or both, is up to you. How can someone make a truly informed decision about treatment if they are not even aware of the existence of alternative therapies? As a licensed medical doctor I am not really allowed to tell you that alternative cancer treatments can be effective. This book contains information that your doctor will not or cannot give you. Like Bob says, "If I had cancer, this is what I would do." Thanks, Bob.

Lynn Jennings, M.D.

FOREWORD THREE

"KILLING CANCER – NOT PEOPLE"

ROBERT (Bob) Wright should receive every accolade and award known to mankind for his literary health work of art, *Killing Cancer – Not People*. This is by far the greatest book written today about your health and staying free from cancer! As a cancer survivor myself – and nutrition advocate – it is with great privilege that I am able to write and let people know, in print, what I have told thousands of people personally about this amazing book.

Up until about five years ago I was a fitness and nutrition expert that companies like Mattel, Xerox, and even Playboy hired for self-defense seminars, kick-boxing and fitness. I didn't do drugs, smoke, or even drink coffee, and took almost every known supplement and herb I read about to stay healthy and disease-free. You can imagine the shock to my system when I found out I had cancer!

I have always strived to be a balanced individual in life, which is always a learning process, intellectually, spiritually, physically, and emotionally. I have been an athlete and practitioner of martial arts for over 35 years now. I participated in forming a 501©(3), non-profit organization that helped kids to stay out of gangs and off drugs and taught them the self-respect and discipline that martial arts provides. I became a therapist over 20 years ago for self-meditation purposes and to assist others with stress, fears, phobias, etc. I have been a city commissioner for two of the cities that I have resided in for the last twelve years and have recently founded a new non-profit organization that addresses the unnecessary deaths of almost 5,000 children per day due to lack of decent drinking water.

So, you ask, how does a seemingly balanced individual that avoids the "bad things in life" – that consumes the right supplements and herbs – get cancer? Good question – and here's the answer. First of all, I bought into everything that I saw on commercials and drank gallons of sports drinks (very acid) that were advertised by all my sports heroes. I "pounded" a literal ton of red meat and other protein because my body building magazine "monsters" told me to. I believed that bottled water was as pure as the mountain stream that it supposedly came from. I used microwave ovens, teflon, and ate my "advertised healthy," low-fat T.V. dinners. I believed everything that doctors and the FDA told me, like a good little sheep.

It wasn't until I got the cancer diagnosis and was literally coerced into radiation treatments for six weeks that I started to do my own due diligence and look for the real truth. I found out about alkalinity and balancing the body pH. I started drinking micro-structured ionized water – full of minerals and anti-oxidants (like Bob addresses in Chapter 6). I immediately dropped 20 pounds and saw family and friends – whom I supplied this water to – have incredible results with diabetes, arthritis, gout, acid reflux, etc.

I have been blessed to be the resident "water expert" at, arguably, the best and healthiest holistic detoxification spa in the world. For twenty-five years now, *We Care Spa* has spread the philosophy of clean and healthy living to people that fly in from all over the world – as well as Hollywood's elite "A" list clientele and health experts. I preach to these very health conscious patrons the brilliance of Bob's book, *Killing Cancer – Not People* – and the word is spreading fast – thank God!

When I was recovering from surgery and radiation, I immersed myself into every health book that was not afraid to tell the real truth about sickness and wellness. I stumbled across *Killing Cancer – Not People* one day and, as I started to read, it was like I had found the "Holy Grail" of health books. This is a no-nonsense book of truth about how, in the last 40 years, we have contributed billions of dollars into research for the disease called cancer and now, mysteriously, more people have cancer and are dying from it than ever before.

Obviously, something is wrong. I can tell you that Bob definitely has the answers – and he has them down to a "science." He speaks the truth – that we are warned by allopathic institutions that alternative medicine is for quacks – but, really, it involves the natural plants, supplements, and treatments that God has provided for us. Bob will give you countless testimonies of people that have been healed using healthy living regimens and not by poisoning their bodies with chemo and radiation.

I am truly honored that Bob has allowed me to put in my two cents worth about his incredible book and implore everyone with cancer – and those of you who never want to get this horrible disease – to pick up, *Killing Cancer – Not People,* and learn the healthy way to a vibrant and cancer-free life!

Thank you, Bob, for all your hard work. You are truly a Godsend.

Chris Young, CHT, City Commissioner
www.watersaveschildren.com

INTRODUCTION

"Darkness cannot drive out darkness — only light can do that."
                    The Reverend Dr. Martin Luther King, Jr.

THERE are literally thousands of books about cancer, its causes, treatments and "cures." One can discover, through these volumes, a myriad of opinions regarding the efficacy of conventional and — the misnamed — "alternative" medical practices.

Of course, only traditional, allopathic (mainstream medicine) measures are licensed and deemed practical protocols for this "malady" that takes up to three-quarters of a million Americans from the face of the earth each year. Think about that for a moment. Every minute of every day someone's mother, father, sister, brother, aunt, uncle, grandparent, spouse or child succumbs to this "non-disease" that is largely preventable. Who will be next? Statistics published on the American Cancer Society Website say one in two men and one in three women — over 40% of us — will have a "cancer experience." Very soon that figure will be a full 50%.

Stand next to someone — one of you will get cancer. I know, I know, you think "it won't be me." Unfortunately, the odds may seem even but they are really against you. Besides, who wants 50-50 odds? I want them to be in my favor — and so should you.

You see, the way we live, what we eat and drink, the environment we exist in, the toxins we ingest — either by choice or chance — these, in large part, are the reasons we get cancer. The so-called experts want you to believe that genetics play a major role. They don't! This is simply not the case. In point of fact, it's estimated that up to 5% of us may carry a gene that pre-disposes us to cancer. And even within this 5%, *the gene must be expressed* to set things in motion. Again, how we live our lives will play a major role in whether or not that "expression" is realized.

The absolute height of folly, ignorance, and tragedy is the fact that women who carry a breast cancer gene – and who have a history of breast cancer in their families – are systematically having both breasts removed as a prophylactic (preventative) measure! And some still get breast cancer in their reconstructed breasts!! *What in the world is going on in this country when a woman, in good health, will allow a surgeon to "cut off" two perfectly good breasts – an action that will change her life forever – to, supposedly, prevent a "disease" that she may, in fact, never get?*

Folks, this is the epitome – no – the "definition" of insanity. In no way do I fault these defenseless women who were talked into this nonsense. They simply did not know the truth. And the truth is (again) that the gene *must be expressed* and, by following the right preventative protocol, the odds are that this will never happen. And, yes, you heard that right.

Ladies, we need to deal with the real causes of cancer. Gentlemen, we must realize and initiate proven preventative measures that will keep each of us, male or female, from becoming a statistic. This process is called personal responsibility.

Fast forward to the highly touted, $3 billion plus, Human Genome Project that President Clinton announced would be "the language that allowed God to create life." Friends, what a disaster and fraud this has been.

The promise was that this program would lead us (the world) to the discovery of all the genetic variations that are the causative factors relating to disease – especially cancer. So, by "sequencing" or "mapping" all of the three billion or so chemical units of the human genome – we'd have the cure. Right? Wrong.

It seems that many of the researchers are spilling the beans here and voicing that this project is really a sell-out and a financial and scientific fraud of epic proportions – designed to forward or encourage "genetic discrimination and eugenics," and they state that any cures resulting from the project are still years away from realization – if they can be realized at all (thanks to M. Thornley, *Natural News* article, August 30, 2010).

Thornley goes on to state that the "critics say the human genome project suffers from a 'genetic determinist paradigm' or a belief that all illness is caused by genes. There is, they argue, no way to connect a gene to a trait – there are too many other environmental and genetic influences. A connection between a particular gene and a condition can only be considered a predisposition, or susceptibility, rather than an isolated, definitive cause."

Let's leave it right there. Enough said. Case closed. So the next time you hear about the great progress and monumental revelations and discoveries of the human genome folly, pass it off "like the idle wind – which you respect not" (thanks to Shakespeare). Then, diligently seek the truth about cancer and all diseases that, in fact, are healable through the human immune system – one of the ***most powerful forces in life and nature.***

So, you ask, what does all of this mumbo jumbo about truth, cancer, genes, genomes, etc., mean to me? In almost all instances, in the proverbial final analysis, the onus points directly at you. It simply means that ***you*** are responsible – nobody else – for your own health and whether cancer manifests itself in your body.

Sadly, we live in a culture that, in many instances, wants to assign blame and does not want to accept responsibility. But you know, by and large, no one forces us to eat and drink the way we do. No one makes us "not exercise." No, we participate in the cause, which means we can also participate in the cure. And once we endorse this reality, this basic truth, we will be on our way to understanding the concepts that surround the prevention and successful treatments for cancer.

That said, there are no absolute guarantees. However, by understanding the basic tenants and truths about cancer, then applying the real proven treatments and protocols, our chance for survival jumps dramatically and exponentially.

This book is about truth. Cancer truth. It is not a "feel good" monologue to help stricken Americans come to terms with their out-of-whack cellular systems (cancer). No, this is real life. This is about cause and effect – the breakdown of the human organism and its resurrection by natural means. No smoke and mirrors here. No false statistics, no unproven theories or bogus "facts." As Joe Friday used to say on "<u>Dragnet</u>," "Just the facts, ma'am." And that's all that you'll find here.

As you meander your way through the following couple of hundred pages, I ask you to think about truth – the very importance of its existence – and what separates it from the "fiction" that life throws at us daily, especially involving cancer. Consider the following quotations as you dwell on life's truths and, particularly, what you know – and will herein discover – is the "real" truth about cancer, its prevention and healing:

"You can bend it and twist it. You can misuse it and abuse it. But even God cannot change the Truth."

Michael Lew

"You never find yourself until you face the truth."

Pearl Bailey

"The truth is incontrovertible. Malice may attack it, ignorance may deride it, but in the end – there it is."

Winston Churchill

"What you perceive, your observations, feelings, interpretations, are all your truth. Your truth is important. Yet it is not The Truth."

Linda Ellinor

"Unthinking respect for authority is the greatest enemy of truth."

Albert Einstein

"Never assume the obvious is true."

William Safire

"The first reaction to truth is hatred."

Tertullian Quotes

"Truth is like the sun. You can shut it out for a time, but it ain't goin' away."

Elvis Presley

"A lie gets half way around the world before the truth has a chance to get its pants on."

Winston Churchill

"If you look for truth, you may find comfort in the end. If you look for comfort, you will not get either comfort or truth – only soft soap and wishful thinking to begin, and in the end, despair."

C.S. Lewis

"The truth, of course, is that a billion falsehoods told a billion times by a billion people – are still false."

Travis Walton

"It is error alone which needs the support of government. Truth can stand by itself."

Thomas Jefferson

"We do not err because truth is difficult to see. It is visible at a glance. We err because this is more comfortable."

Alexander Solzhenitsyn

This work strives to cover ground not addressed by most other cancer literature. If you acquire this deadly *disease* (many don't believe it is a disease under the strict definition), what do you do? This book is about **exactly** what I would do if I had cancer – and from that point forward, with a cancer diagnosis – it would be my cancer treatment guide. Whether it becomes yours, or not, is entirely up to you.

We are trained to go to the doctor when we believe something is wrong. I am not suggesting for a moment that you don't do precisely that. When I grew up, God was placed at the highest level in our lives – no one and nothing trumped God. And the family doctor resided just slightly under the Almighty. That's how incredibly much the "Doc" was honored and respected. As a result, we did exactly what he or she said – no wavering, no questions, no debate.

However, being a more educated populace with access to resources far beyond what our ancestors enjoyed, it's long past time to question. Let me clarify that statement. Good doctors, hospitals, nurses and other medical practitioners are vital and necessary. If I get into a car crash and am seriously injured, I want the best surgeon, anesthesiologist and other medical staff that money can buy. These trained and educated professionals are a lifesaving requirement in our society, when needed.

Therein lies the "rub." Allopathic medicine has evolved far beyond its level of expertise. And I know that your next question is "just what the heck does that mean?" It means, simply, that all medical personnel and experts have a role to play and a function to serve. While doctors are trained in disease, diagnostics and drugs (the alliteration of conventionality in medicine), they study very little about nutrition and how the body reacts and responds to nutrients, water, vitamins, minerals and natural supplements. Just ask a doctor – he or she will verify that their course of study included but a few hours (or less) on nutrition! What's a phytonutrient? Where would you find one, what do they do? None of this information is a part of standard medical school curriculum.

There's the problem. We trust our doctors (and pharmaceuticals) to heal us when they really have no ability to do so. Contrary to popular belief (and hope), drugs don't heal people and neither do doctors. Your very own body, in fact, has been endowed by The Creator with an amazing weapon – the human immune system. If functioning properly and treated with adequate nutrition, it has the innate ability to heal virtually *anything* thrown at it, and that includes cancer. And, no, this is not an essay about nutrition – although it plays the most important role in whether or not you survive cancer.

This book is a guide – it is comprised of exactly what I would do if I had cancer. I have studied alternative medicine, supplements and protocols, the cancer industry, traditional medicine, statistics, and the science and treatment of cancer for years. By the grace of God, I have been able to discover the **real truth** about cancer; it's causes, prevention and treatments. And these are the treatments that have proven, time and time again, over decades of use by real people, to actually **work.**

Don't be fooled. Chemotherapy, radiation and surgery cannot heal you – although surgery is sometimes absolutely necessary. Sometimes. We will address this further in Chapter 2.

If you contract cancer – if you have it right now – you want only the truth and the facts about how you can heal. That's what this book is about and it explains exactly what I would do if I was diagnosed with this disease.

The protocols herein have proven effective for literally tens of thousands of people – just like you and me – who chose to forgo the cut, burn and poison conventions, or who had already gone through these, only to be sent home to die. The truth is – natural therapies and treatments work – traditional measures usually do not. And that's a fact.

Conventional wisdom and conventional medicine may well be furious with the "unmitigated gall" that I must possess to publish such a "blatant falsehood" regarding the treatment of cancer. I am not moved. My motivation lies in the healed bodies of multitudes of cancer sufferers who are walking around and thriving today because they did the *right thing* – not the *usual and customary thing.* There is no satisfaction and no consolation in the latter when your family hears "we did the best we could." And, the truth be known, most of us are aware, deep down, that the result is usually always the same – the patient "didn't survive."

Truth. Nothing but the truth. No, I won't present to you anything that doesn't have pure facts behind it. There will be no attempt to convince you to try something because, in a clinical trial, only four people died and nobody seemed to get any worse. There will be no forwarding of drugs that killed some cancer cells in lab rats. I won't insult anybody's intelligence by saying that everything that is promoted in this book will cure them.

Rather, as I ask all mainstream research clinicians, institutions, medical doctors and drug companies to show me the plain, unadulterated facts and truth behind their studies and treatments that don't appear to bear fruit or assist cancer sufferers, I will show you the "empirical evidence," the real truth about what works to heal cancer. My Great Hekawi (Ha-cow-ee) Grandmother used to say, "the proof is in the pudding." I believed her then – I believe her now. Test the pudding, folks. Make sure it's edible, palatable, and good.

What you will read in this book is patient-proven and time-tested. A literal library of testimonies shouts out the healing proficiency of the treatments, therapies, and protocols forwarded herein. But you must put it to the test. Do your own homework and investigation. Prove it to yourself. And after you have done that, get to work on it, cancer or not. I ask you to always keep at the forefront of your thoughts the concept that what heals cancer also prevents it; and what prevents cancer also heals it. When you think about it – it makes perfect sense.

It's now up to you. My suggestion – go for it! That's what I would do.

"The ultimate aim of the human mind, in all its efforts, is to become acquainted with Truth."
                    Eliza Farnham, American Reformer (1815-1864)

"The truth is out there."
                                        Fox Mulder, *The X-Files*

CHAPTER ONE

"CANCER: WHERE WE ARE AND WHY WE'RE HERE"

"However, if a doctor tells a patient that cancer can be cured by means of blood and tissue detox, and offers to provide such a cure, they are likely to be prosecuted. It is not 'politically correct' these days for doctors to discuss the real causes of cancer, nor to provide real cures that work, because the profits of powerful pharmaceutical cartels and other branches of the modern medical industry are threatened by the truth regarding the real causes and cures for disease."

Daniel Reid – "*The Tao of Detox*"

MY father took his last breath at 4:02 a.m., September 24th, 2008. I know, I was there in the half-light of his apartment bedroom. It was an awful thing to witness. He had suffered for years with chronic kidney failure and lung disease. One cancerous kidney had been removed a dozen years prior and this lurking killer had been moving on to the other one. Continuous dialysis, lung drainage by syringe, and 24 prescription drugs for everything from constipation to high blood pressure and pain had haunted his last several years. Finally, he gave up.

I'm sure that a similar story is shared among many American families today. In one way or another, we all have been touched by the plague of cancer. The number one killer of Dads and Moms, brothers, sisters and children today is the "Big C." I'm here to tell you it shouldn't be so.

Look back for a moment to the turn of the 20th Century. Yes, that "way back" era when the average person ate whole foods spawned from mineral-rich soils, uncontaminated by gallons of inorganic pesticides. A wistful time when a piece of candy or a soda pop was a rare treat – not a multi-daily occurrence. Trans fats were unheard of, hydrogenated oils were yet to come, high-fructose corn syrup was non-existent, there was still iodine in our bread, and the average "Joe" consumed only 5 pounds of sugar yearly instead of the *170 pounds* we ingest today. Those "good 'ol days" are long gone.

No, the diet wasn't perfect back then, but it reflected the body's need for plant nutrients (remember vegetables?), fresh fruits, whole grains and nuts, and unadulterated meats and dairy products. No need to tell you that these types of foods are generally absent from the average dietary protocol of today. They have been replaced with burgers, shakes, fries (aren't they a vegetable?), soda pop, artificial sweeteners, margarine, flavor enhancers, preservatives, and processed foods of every form. It has become increasingly evident that the food we eat *is killing us*.

We take showers in highly chlorinated water (chlorine is poison); we drink water with fluoride (fluoride is poison) and chlorine in it; we use deodorants with chemicals and aluminum in them; we smoke cigarettes with over 100 known carcinogens; we stopped exercising; we sit on our proverbial butts watching television, playing video games, talking on cell phones, etc., etc., etc. Tell me, is it any wonder we get sick?

When we are born, our bodies are slightly alkaline and, in most instances, this produces a very healthy inner environment. From that point forward, however, we seem to do everything possible to change the alkaline terrain in our bodies to acidic. Literally, and largely because of what we consume, we start "rotting" from the inside out.

Ever smell a newborn baby? Smells good – alkaline. Ever walk into a nursing home? Smells bad – acid. For those who haven't caught on yet, alkaline is good, acid is bad. Alkaline is healthy, acid is sickness. It's simply a fact. I believe that acidosis is the basic cause of most or all disease known to man. Do you remember the pH (potential of hydrogen) scale back in high school? It's a logarithmic scale from 0 to 14 with 7 being neutral. Everything below that is acid, above is alkaline. Every jump of 1 point (like the seismic Richter Scale) is 10 times the preceding value. An alkaline reading of 8.5 is 10 times more alkaline than one of 7.5. Likewise, a body with a pH of 4.5 (diseased) is 100 times more acidic than one with a pH of 6.5 (10 X 10). Get the picture? Incredibly, the urine pH of many cancer patients is in the 4 range. And **all** cancer patients are acidic!

In his book entitled *The Seven Pillars of Health,* Dr. Don Colbert, M.D., says, "In an alkaline environment your tissues get rid of impurities more efficiently. When cancer patients come into my office to begin nutritional treatment, their bodies are almost always very acidic and toxic. My first task is to get their tissues to alkalinize with alkaline water and alkaline foods."

Regarding how acid and oxygen play into the cancer scenario, Dr. Bruce West condenses it for us in plain English:

"And while we are at it, you need to know that probably everyone over age 50 has cancer of one sort or another somewhere in their body at any given time. Most will never know it because their body will simply cure it. These are the survivors. And they are the strong people – ones with a strong immune system who – whether they know they have a cancer or not, and with or without drugs, surgery or radiation – maintain a strong immune system, strong spirit, and strong mind to beat cancer.

"You can be one of these millions of people, once you know that cancer thrives in an *acidic, anaerobic (without oxygen), toxic, and immune-weakened environment in your body.* Therefore, taking steps to maintain a proper acid/alkaline balance, increase oxygen levels, decrease toxin levels or detoxify the body, and strengthen the immune system are the keys to preventing cancer. And while this sounds daunting, it is not only easy, it can become a way of life – one that will make you feel better, younger, and provide benefits to your health – no matter what problems plague you, including cancer."

Simply put, what we eat, what we drink, what we put on and in our bodies, what we breathe, how we move (exercise) or don't move, either makes us sick or keeps us well. And while there are rare exceptions, this is truth, this is fact, whether or not you agree – and whether you like it or not.

President Richard Nixon declared war on cancer in 1971, authorizing multi-millions of dollars to rid the United States of this scourge. Gee, by my calculations that was *four decades* ago and yet, today, more people get cancer and suffer immeasurably from non-working, unproven conventional treatments – then die from it – than ever before. What could possibly have happened?

We have now spent literally trillions (with a "t") of dollars for research, drugs and treatments, with absolutely nothing to show for it. There are now more people working in the "cancer industry" than actually have cancer! And there is no shortage of cancer patients. The saddest and most tragic part of all of this is that we're not only dying of the "disease" now, we're dying from the *treatments* (more in Chapter 2).

While I don't subscribe to conspiracy theory nor am I interested in politicizing this fact, the truth is that cancer is about money and power. And remember, this book is about truth – not hearsay, not theory, not baseless conjecture – just the truth. There are many who declare that the American Cancer Society is the largest and most corrupt non-profit organization on the planet. With a budget in the billions, additional billions of dollars of assets (a non-profit?), and almost three-quarters of a century of existence, tell me, *where are the cures?* Wouldn't you think that any entity with those kinds of resources, that was seriously and truly looking for a cure for cancer, would have found one by now?

The fact is – through never-ending conventional methodologies, drugs and research – we are almost exactly where we were 40 years ago. Let's face it; there is no money in a cure for cancer. And cancer **_cannot_** be cured with drugs, surgery, chemo or radiation; not now, not ever, not possible. So where, you might ask, have all those billions (or trillions) of dollars for "the cure" actually gone? They have gone the way of the flowers, "gone to graveyards, every one" – and, to continue that song, "when will they ever learn, when will they ever learn?" Actually, I like to say that all those hard-earned, tax-payer dollars have disappeared into the huge, black, sucking hole that is called **_"cancer research"_** – never to be seen or heard from again. Harsh – but accurate. And just so you don't think that Bob is off on a wild tangent at this point, filled with emotion and spouting unproven theories or "fantasy facts," listen to what these well-schooled, infinitely-researched and studied experts have to say on this subject.

First, let's hear from well respected (and somewhat irreverent – you've got to love this guy), Dr. William Campbell Douglass, M.D:

"Here's what October smells like: burning leaves, pumpkin pie, and B.S. That's because it's Breast Cancer Awareness Month, which is practically a national holiday at this point. And if you don't join the 'in' crowd and slap a pink ribbon on whatever you're wearing, you're treated like some kind of cold-blooded, breast-hating monster.

"But those pink ribbons don't exist to cure disease or save lives – they represent a Big Pharma-funded effort to drive millions of women through a funnel of screenings for a disease many don't even have, and treatments that most of them don't even need. In fact, the supposed benefits of all those screenings and treatments are about as real as the Great Pumpkin – and the numbers prove it every time.

"Breast Cancer Awareness Month is now 26 years old. In the 26 years since it was launched by AstraZeneca to help sell the company's cancer drugs, it's been a wild success – for AstraZeneca and anyone else who makes money off cancer screenings and treatments. But when it comes to saving lives and curing disease, it's been a miserable failure. Up to 15 lives are ruined with unnecessary and deforming breast-chopping surgeries and poisonous radiation treatments for every life 'saved.' And even then, there's no guarantee that the one life 'saved' was actually the result of early detection and brutal mainstream treatments – because plenty of them were actually CAUSED by the radioactive and tumor-bursting screenings in the first place."

And listen to this next quotation from world-famous aspartame researcher, Betty Martini:

"In the early 90's, my friend Michelle and I walked with these ladies. I had thousands of copies made of a speech I had given at the Capital on the cure for cancer and, of course, aspartame information – original studies showed more mammary tumors than brain tumors. The representatives there were furious and asked us to leave. I told them it was public property and they were out of luck. Michelle said, 'Do you really want to cure breast cancer or are you in it for bigger bonuses and money?' She answered, 'We want the money, *we're not interested in the cure,* now leave!' I never forgot that."

Finally, from the ever-vigilant, tell-it-like-it-really-is, Health Ranger, Mike Adams, wrap your arms around this:

"The 'Race for the Cure' is one of the greatest sociomedical cons ever pulled off by the pharmaceutical industry. Here's how it works: First, the drug companies take over the cancer non-profits by donating huge sums of money and getting their own executives on the boards of these organizations. From there, all decisions by the cancer non-profits are made to protect the interests of drug companies. Today, virtually all cancer non-profits are actually Big Pharma front groups that push cancer treatment, but never prevention (because actually preventing cancer would harm the profits of drug companies).

"Next, these cancer front groups pull off a double-whammy con job by first convincing people that money is the only obstacle to finding a 'cure' for cancer. Then they convince people to actually hand over money for the right to run around in circles so they can feel like they're helping to find this so-called cure.

"Cancer, you see, is big, big business. And keeping that money flowing requires a global propaganda campaign that holds out a carrot of hope in order to keep all the 'sheeple' running in circles, emptying their pockets of cash for the benefit of the drug companies. The scale of this scam is astounding."

Astounding, indeed. Friends, you just can't make this stuff up. Money and power, much to our dismay and chagrin, are the drivers behind this powerful and corrupt cancer industry.

Those of you in North Carolina may have seen the Morehead City *News Times* article on January 10th, 2010, that revealed the following startling revelation:

"Vernon Hill, a successful 'Relay for Life' volunteer leader who had raised nearly nine hundred thousand dollars ($900,000) for the American Cancer Society, resigned after his Internet research found that high ranking officers of the ACS were making as much as a million dollars a year with benefits, like a company car and lucrative pensions. He also found that a very small percentage of the money goes to actual research.

"The same network of cancer causers and cancer profiteers has ruled the war on cancer for 40 years. For the most part, their only successes have been in fattening their pockets and in creating a system that prevents research and treatments which could make a difference. The sooner the public wakes up to the truth about the failed war on cancer and the organizations which have become a part of the problem instead of the solution, the sooner we will be able to realize true cancer prevention and lasting cures."

Ladies and gentlemen, there is no money in the things that actually enable the human body to heal itself, whether it be food, natural supplements, therapeutic, non-invasive therapies and treatments or baking soda. Those who have dared to challenge the status quo of treatments and research have been ridiculed, tarred and feathered and run out of town on a rail, sent to prison, financially ruined – and WORSE: Harry Hoxsey, Royal Raymond Rife, Jason Vale – to name just a few – and every doctor, clinic, or researcher who has been chased to Mexico by the FDA and the FTC for "healing" cancer patients through "unapproved" devices, foods, natural supplements, et al. How dare they buck the system! They've got their nerve!

I appreciate and admire those who raise money for cancer research. For the most part, they do it for all the right reasons. They have suffered or have a family member or friend who has. Their motives are pure and they deserve great credit for trying desperately to fund a "cure." Unfortunately, the majority cannot tell you where the money they raise or donate ends up. When asked, most will answer "cancer research." Somehow, that "stock" reply seems sufficient for them. If this is you – or if this were me – I would want to know (nay, *demand* to know) that my hard earned dollars – or dollars raised through great effort – were really making a difference. Sadly, most are not. Next time – question! Discover the truth. Raise money for, or give your dollars to, an organization that is doing the right thing for cancer patients. Please, for the expedited arrival of the "real" cure, *just do it* (thank you Nike).

So, this is where we are – and this is how we got here (the short version). Personally and individually, most of us are doing the wrong things by eating the wrong foods, living lives largely devoid of real nutrition, adequate hydration and exercise and, instead, filling our swelling bodies with poisons, toxins, proton-pump inhibitors and sugar – then wondering why we have acid reflux and cancer (and all other diseases). And when all is said and done, we seem to be O.K. with that. We spend 40, 50, 60 years becoming acid and obese with the never-ending hope and belief that our doctor (revered just slightly below God) will produce the magic pill that will take off the pounds and heal us.

Sadly, in real life, it doesn't work that way. Once again, the truth is that conventional medical science and practice have no answers for you – especially with cancer. Nor will they – ever – at their current rate of producing "cures." Sure, they can diagnose and utilize allopathic measures for symptoms. Yes, they can call your sickness "chronic" and, virtually, treat you to death (and, if you let them, they will). But they cannot heal you. Only your body itself can do that. However, you must do the right things and undertake the proper plan to make that happen.

Dr. Jimmy Steger, one of America's great Naturopathic Doctors and Clinical Nutritionists, with a thriving practice (actually, he doesn't practice – he knows what he's doing) in Mobile, Alabama, tells us exactly "where we are – and why we're here" through his summation of *The American Death Ceremony*. Sit back – you're going to enjoy this:

"The American Death Ceremony started as a ritual back in the days of witchcraft. The last few years it has been developed into a science. It usually takes from fifteen to twenty years. However, modern scientific advancements are shortening this period of time.

"It starts with one simple pain relieving aspirin for a simple headache or backache. When one aspirin will no longer mask the pain, then you decide to take two. After a few months, when two aspirin will no longer mask the pain in the head or back, you take a stronger compound. By this time it becomes necessary to take something for the ulcers in your stomach that have been caused by the aspirin. Now we have two medicines in our body, and you have a great start.

"After a few months, these medications are starting to disrupt your liver function. If a good infection develops, you now take some penicillin. Of course, penicillin will damage your red blood corpuscles and spleen so that you develop anemia. Another medication is then taken to cover up the anemia. By the time all of these medications put such a strain on your kidneys – they should break down.

"It's now time to introduce some antibiotics into the system. When these destroy your natural resistance to disease, you can expect a general flair-up of all your symptoms. The next important step is to cover up all of these symptoms with some good sulfur-based drugs. When the kidneys finally plug up you can have them drained. Some poison will build up in your system, but you can keep going quite a while this way.

"By now the medications in your body will be so confused they won't know what they are supposed to be doing, but it really doesn't matter. If you have followed every step as directed by your family physician, you can now make an appointment with your undertaker.

"This game is played by practically all Americans in this country, except for the few ignorant souls who follow nature's way.

"Drugs only mask the symptoms allowing the body, at best, time to heal itself. We must give our body the tools that are necessary to rebuild and regenerate healthy cells. These are minerals such as copper, calcium, magnesium, iodine, manganese, zinc, potassium, cobalt, sodium, selenium, and chromium. Without these elemental minerals in the body, you will not make it to see sixty or seventy years of age. These minerals, taken on a daily basis through our diets and through additional supplementation, will allow our bodies to rebuild their own internal bio-magnetic energy form. We are then capable of pulling out of our food source those additional minerals our bodies deem necessary for proper health."

Many will not want to believe this but, in most cases, without this natural, non-chemical plan, you are lost. Your body *will* heal itself only if you treat it right and give it what it needs (and really craves). While there are many different "alternative" anti-cancer, healing protocols that have proven effective, this book will show you what I would do if I were told I had cancer. For many, this plan and similar natural therapies have made the difference between healing – or not.

Read, study, and digest this information. After that – it's up to you.

CHAPTER TWO

"THE BIG THREE: SURGERY, CHEMOTHERAPY, AND RADIATION – JUST THE FACTS, MA'AM"

"Another disturbing fact about chemotherapy is that the majority of specialists who prescribe such drugs would refuse to take them if they or their families had cancer themselves. According to one study published in the 'Journal of Clinical Oncology' in 1987, 81% of cancer specialists would not consent to a drug trial due to the ineffectiveness of chemotherapy and its unacceptable degree of toxicity."

Zohan Rona, M.D. – *The Failure of Chemotherapy*

SLASH, POISON, BURN. The Big Three. You probably know them better as surgery, chemotherapy and radiation. What you probably don't know is that they have no possibility of healing your cancer. Let me repeat that. They have *absolutely no* possibility of healing your cancer. They actually *cause* cancer.

Traditional oncology has a fascination with tumors. The logic appears to be that "if we get that thing out of there the cancer will go away." And I've got some cheap beachfront property for sale in eastern Nebraska . ....

Let me say (nay, shout) to you right here and now what all "alternative medicine" practitioners, researchers and educators know for a fact

– and please remember this: *a tumor is only a symptom of a deeper problem; it is the body's method of encapsulating the invader, the cancer. If you take it out, the cancer is still there.* But day after day, week after week, year after year, surgery is performed in every hospital in America to "remove the tumor" – that symptom of a cellular malfunction that has been growing and expanding in your body for more than five or ten years. And, in most instances, the cancer (tumor) comes back with a vengeance because "the big three" don't deal with the actual cause of the problem. And, once that has happened, once it is "back" (it actually never left), it is now more difficult than ever to kill – even through alternative methodologies.

If you have a cancerous tumor (or tumors) and you are still upright and mobile, without much pain, and are able to carry on your daily routine, you simply do not have enough cancer to kill you. Did you get that? So, if you could stop the tumor(s) from growing at that moment, couldn't you virtually continue your normal life and live with it? Of course, you wouldn't want to do that – but you actually could.

Modern medicine, with all its wonderful new diagnostic equipment, surgical techniques and drugs, would have you believe that the tumor is the cancer and if you don't get it out right now you are done. Not true on both counts. The tumor is a symptom and you almost always have time. If you don't believe this last sentence – here's what generally happens: first, you are frightened into believing that surgery and chemical/radiological treatments are your only chance and you must start right now and, second, you are scheduled for surgery, cut open and cut up, told "we got it all" (they never get it all), then set up for chemo and radiation. Your demise has begun.

You are told nothing of alternative therapies and, in many instances, threatened if you even consider them. Please understand, however, that if your Doctor knew of any "non-traditional, natural cancer treatments, he could lose his medical license should he tell you about, or recommend, any of these treatments – the treatments that could actually save your life. If you follow this allopathic regimen and begin the poison/burn protocol – your chances of survival are immediately and significantly diminished. Your immune system, already stressed by surgery, will suffer major damage (or destruction) through these radical introductions at a time when you actually need it to be as strong as possible.

Poison, radiation and surgery cannot heal you. I know, I know. How can this "pillar" of the American Community (the much beloved Doctor) possibly be wrong? How can he/she be promoting something that won't help me (or, in fact, will hurt me)? Good questions – both.

Well, here are the facts – and here is the truth. When it comes to cancer, your traditional doctor/oncologist will fail you and almost all cancer sufferers miserably. And statistics prove it. Despite what you may have heard from the American Cancer Society and its minions, only 3% (or less) of those undergoing conventional treatments (chemo) survive for five years. Fact – not fiction. These stats were published in the December 2004 issue of *Clinical Oncology* by Morgan, Ward, and Barton and they present these results: "*The overall contribution of curative and adjuvant cytotoxic chemotherapy to 5-year survival in adults was estimated to be 2.3% in Australia and 2.1% in the USA.*"

German biostatistician and epidemiologist, Ulrich Abel, contacted over 350 medical centers around the world in the 1980's requesting them to furnish him with anything they had published on the subject of cancer. By the time he finished his report in 1990, he was said to know more about chemotherapy than anyone. His report described chemo as a "scientific wasteland" and that neither physician nor patient were willing to give up even though there was no scientific evidence that it worked. *Geeeeeez.*

And think about this for a moment. If a patient dies during a chemo study, he is eliminated from the statistics because he did not complete the study! Those darn quitters, anyway.

This is truth, backed by scientific, epidemiological studies and documentation that are not subject to question or debate. And while I'm sure that it is not what America wants to hear or what allopathic medicine wants published – it's true, nonetheless.

Want more proof? Ph.D. Ralph Moss, who is a former Director of Information for Sloan Kettering Cancer Research Center (boy, there's another story), says that "chemotherapy is basically ineffective in the vast majority of cases in which it is given." Dr. Moss continues by adding that "conventional cancer therapy is so toxic and dehumanizing that I fear it far more than I fear death from cancer. We know that conventional therapy doesn't work – if it did, you would not fear cancer any more than you fear pneumonia. It is the utter lack of certainty as to the outcome of conventional treatment that virtually screams for more freedom of choice in the area of cancer therapy. Yet, most alternative therapies, regardless of potential or proven benefit, are outlawed, which forces patients to submit to the failures that we know don't work, because there's no other choice."

Dr. Julian Whitaker, M.D., purports that "I wouldn't have chemotherapy and radiation because I'm not interested in therapies that cripple the immune system and, in my opinion, virtually ensure failure for the majority of cancer patients."

Dr. Gary Null, Ph.D., speaks of a listener to his radio show in the following excerpt:

"I have a doctor who called me last year. He listens to the show and personally he lives a healthy life. And he was angry. And he didn't know what to do. He wanted to know whether or not he could expose the situation without getting himself involved. He said, 'I'm giving cancer patients over here at this major cancer clinic drugs that are killing them, and I can't stop it because they said the protocol's what's important.' And I say, 'But the patient's not doing well.' They say, 'The protocol's what's important, not the patient.' And he said, 'You can't believe what goes on in the name of medicine and science in this country.'"

Dr. Tullio Simoncini – or as many of us know him – the "cancer is a fungus/sodium bicarbonate physician," is having great success with simple baking soda in killing cancer cells. Dr. Simoncini lays it on the line regarding chemotherapy in this missive:

"Chemotherapy, in fact, destroys everything. It is a given fact that it dramatically exhausts the cells of the marrow and of the blood, thus allowing a greater spreading of the infection. It irreversibly intoxicates the liver, thus preventing it from building new elements of defense, and it mercilessly knocks out nerve cells, thus weakening the organism's reactive capabilities and delivering it to the invaders. This is mainly because it is not clear how it affects the colonies and, because by strongly debilitating the organism, such intervention makes the invasion of the mycetes (fungus) faster and more ferocious."

Author of *Thousand Plants Against Cancer Without Chemotherapy*, Dr. Giuseppe Nacci, M.D., gets to the bottom of chemo statistics:

"Very often, the simple truth is absolutely not believed; you can recover from cancer but not from chemotherapy. Out of fifty people suffering from cancer who decide to undergo chemotherapy, only one will still be alive after only five years from the first chemotherapy cycle."

Dr. Sam Epstein goes on record declaring that "chemotherapy and radiation can increase the risk of developing a second cancer by up to ***100 times***" (emphasis mine). According to Dr. Martin Shapiro of UCLA, "Cancer researchers, medical journals, and the popular media all have contributed to a situation in which many people with common malignancies are being treated with drugs not known to be effective." Dr. Albert Braverman wrote in the *Lancet* that "many medical oncologists recommend chemotherapy for virtually any tumor, with a hopefulness undiscouraged by almost invariable failure."

And Dr. Tim O'Shea minces no words when he emphatically states this:

> "Cytotoxic is the word that describes chemotherapeutic drugs. It means 'cell-killing.' Chemotherapy kills all the cells of the body, not just the cancer cells. The risk is that chemo will kill the patient before it kills the cancer – which usually happens. Therefore, the only question that should be asked when deciding whether or not to begin chemo is this: will this drug prolong the patient's natural lifespan? Is it likely to? The unadorned data says no."

Believe it or not, most Americans today believe that chemotherapy is safe and that it, along with radiation, are the only proven treatments for cancer. Mike Adams, the Health Ranger, states that "chemotherapy is a fraud, plain and simple. Chemotherapy causes vomiting, hair loss, muscle loss, brain damage, heart damage, kidney damage, and liver damage. Much of this damage is permanent."

Somebody, please stop me. In reality, the quotes – representing the real *"facts"* regarding chemotherapy – could fill several large books.

And, how about that radiation therapy? Professor John Cairns, from the Harvard University School of Public Health, said in 1985, "The majority of cancers cannot be cured by radiation because the dose of X-rays required to kill all the cancer cells would also kill the patient."

Dr. Robert R. Jones, said in 1980, "Many radiation complications do not occur for several years after treatment, giving the therapist and the patient a false sense of security for a year or two following therapy…the bone marrow, in which blood cells are made, is largely obliterated in the field of irradiation…This is an irreversible effect."

Dr. Lucien Israel, consultant to the NCI, reported in 1978 that "people who undergo radiation therapy are more likely to have their cancer metastasize to other sites." Other studies have supported this view. He also stated that "the radioactivity intended to kill cancer cells can, instead, trigger mutations that create new cancer cells of other types." (Radiation quotes from the www.starthealthylife.com site).

From *Empty Harvest*, by Dr. Bernard Jenson and Mark Anderson, comes this:

"British physician Alice Steward has spent much of her life investigating the connection between low-level radiation and higher cancer risks. Most doctors have stopped using fetal x-rays since Stewart's work showed that a significant increase in leukemia was found in the children of mothers who had prenatal x-rays taken. She has said she believes that the effects of background radiation coupled with exposure to x-rays may cause most childhood cancer."

Cause and effect. Radiation causing cancer, radiation spreading cancer, radiation killing patients – the entire package accompanied by the whole nine yards.

Timothy Brantley's, *The Cure: Heal Your Body, Save Your Life,* causes us pause with this assessment:

"If this process was safe and effective for someone who was in remission, then why didn't they give radiation to everyone, just to make sure cancer never attacked them? Why didn't the doctors, their wives, and their children take radiation as a preventative measure? I pictured a radiation drive-thru like a fast-food window.

They literally fried my mother's chest with what I would later discover was an enormous amount of radiation therapy. When I saw the radiation burns on my mother's chest, I wondered if no treatment at all would have been a better bet."

And the answer to that last query is an unqualified "yes."

You know, I could go on and on. I could recite statistics and list quotes about the lack of effectiveness of all three of these mainstream treatments. I think you get the point. The purpose of this book is not to go deep about what causes cancer or to fill you with evidence of the failure of conventional medicine. If you want more of this, buy a copy of Ty Bollinger's *Cancer – Step Outside the Box.* Ty gives a more in-depth study of chemo, surgery and radiation therapy and has loads of quotation documentation. His book is an excellent source for cancer data and conspiracy. Actually, you don't have to look very long or very hard to find scores of white papers, journal reviews, and books about the true and utter failure of conventional medicine when it comes to cancer treatments and therapies.

I believe that it is important to note, at this point, that conventional oncological medicine should really be the medical sector of treatment branded as "alternative." There is no evidence that these treatments either heal or help – and plenty of evidence and documentation that they will actually hurt you – or worse. What happened to "first, do no harm?" The real "conventional medicine" should be the non-lethal, immune system building, natural supplement, non-toxic therapies and protocols that have stood the test of time and have allowed the human body to heal itself. Although not proven by FDA supported "clinical trials" – that are only allowed for Pharmaceutical Companies and prove nothing – these protocols have produced volumes of well-documented, empirical evidence (through hundreds of thousands of healed bodies) that is overwhelming, statistically impressive, and undeniable. Jerry McGuire and the local hospital may say, "Show me the money." Those who know the real facts and statistics about cancer will "show you the truth."

This chapter was meant to be brief. You need to know **what to do** about your cancer – or that of a loved one. So let's proceed and I will tell you what I would do if I had cancer. But before we move on – let me say this unequivocally: I would **never** undergo chemotherapy or radiation treatments because they do not heal, they are devastating to the body, and they actually cause cancer. And I would not undergo surgery unless it was absolutely and imminently necessary to save my life. Period. You must, however, make your own decisions regarding these traditional cancer interventions. But base them on fact, personal investigation and truth – not the will or forcefulness of a conventionally trained doctor or oncologist. It's your life – not his – take charge of it.

Educate yourself concerning the "real truth" about cancer. Actually strive to know more than your cancer doctor. It's not that difficult since most know only "The Big Three." You'll be forever grateful that you undertook this task – and so will your family – for years to come.

CHAPTER THREE

"WHAT YOU MUST DO FIRST – WHAT YOU MUST STOP DOING RIGHT NOW"

"Tragically, that means we're not just dumping toxic fluoride into our drinking water. We're also exposing innocent, unsuspecting people to deadly elements of lead, arsenic, and radium, all of them carcinogenic. Because of the cumulative properties of toxins, the detrimental effects on human health are catastrophic."

Dr. Hardy Limeback, Ph.D., Biochemistry,
D.D.S., Department of Preventative Dentistry,
University of Toronto

DAVE'S STORY

SOME time ago, I stopped in to see my friend Dave who had recently been diagnosed with colon cancer. Several months earlier he had passed some blood in his stool and was concerned enough to see his doctor and schedule a colonoscopy. The subsequent test report showed a rather large tumor in his descending colon and a CT scan revealed four half-dollar sized faint images on his liver. In layman's terms, the cancer had spread (metastasized).

After all the tests were complete, he finally got to see the oncologist. I asked him what the doctor told him. Dave's response – "He told me I was gonna die." He went on to say that the doc gave him "up to" eighteen months if he hit the chemo hard and only about six months, or less, if he did nothing. In other words, he gave him nothing to hope for – save a few extra months of a "low quality" existence if he chose conventional treatments.

I believe that if you want to expedite the demise of cancer patients – tell them that they have no hope. And if they buy into that prognosis, they will expire rapidly. If they don't – and fight – they actually have a chance. We will address this issue further in Chapter Nine.

After much consultation, Dave initially chose to start on a natural, non-surgical, non-chemical, non-radiological protocol involving an alkaline diet and water, detoxification, and supplementation designed to oxygenate and alkalinize his cells. He was on the right track. Within four to six weeks he appeared to be doing better and his "Navarro Urine Test" (see "Cancer Testing" later in this chapter) had gone down a point – revealing cancer remission. About two weeks later – it happened. He was rushed to the hospital with excruciating pain under his right rib cage (liver).

Upon examination, it was determined that he was severely dehydrated and nurses began to hang bag after bag of saline solution to, literally, "bring him back." You see, Dave hadn't been drinking anything during the previous week, save a sip on a sugar-laden soda pop occasionally. He also wasn't following his detoxing protocol. His body was killing cancer cells but had no way to proficiently eliminate the subsequent debris through the normal process. His major detoxification organ, the liver, was involved in his disease – as is the case with virtually all cancer patients – and not functioning properly. His unwillingness to ingest sufficient fluids compounded his problem.

Dave survived this incident but then, with the help of his doctor, decided that this "natural" protocol was too hard and chemotherapy would be much easier, more effective, would be done *for* him (easy), he could eat whatever he wanted (easy, with "comfort foods"), and he was essentially "oncologist convinced" that he would have a better quality of life for whatever time he had left. Excuse me – but what a crock.

You probably have guessed what happened from that point forward. Round after round of chemo ensued. I asked Dave when he would be finished and he replied, "Never." He went downhill rapidly. I visited him several times during the next few months and he looked worse each time. Eventually, he could no longer get out of his chair, he was thin and pale, very confused, and had trouble communicating. A couple of weeks later, the call came from his son: his Dad had passed. I was deeply saddened – my friend was gone. He had entrusted his *life* to those who literally had no chance to heal him – and no stake in his survival. And, no, he didn't even come close to the promised 18 months.

Unfortunately, this tragedy is repeated many times every day in this country and throughout the world. A cancer patient dies **every minute** in America – and most have undergone our "gold standard" of conventional treatments. And more and more it has become evident that the cancer didn't kill them – the treatment did.

Well, you ask, what does this have to do with "what you must do first and what you must stop doing right now?" Obviously, I can't and won't tell you not to see your doctor. Nor will I ever get between a patient and his or her oncologist. And even though I know that they are ineffective against cancer, are severely debilitating, and can cause your death – I won't tell you to forgo surgery, chemo or radiation treatments. What I can tell you is that I would never subject myself to these proven killers (see Chapter Two). Yes, you may survive – and some do. But long term, most do not. And if they do survive initially, the cancer comes back again and again, stronger and more virulent each time – until the end. It's just not worth it. The fact is that you will survive just as long if you do absolutely nothing. Legitimate studies have proven this. And you will have a better quality of life – no question.

So what you ***must do first***, at the very beginning of this process, is to seriously question traditional treatments and find out the truth about what they are, what they do, and what the real chances of survival are using these methods. What you ***must stop*** doing immediately is closing your eyes and ears to the many proven "alternative" treatments, therapies, protocols and supplements that, most often, make the difference between life and death for a cancer patient.

As the late, great Paul Harvey used to say, "And now – the rest of the story." Let's get to the "must stops" and "must starts" as these need to begin right away if you are to be successful. Please keep in mind that I would pursue the following advice whether I had cancer or not. Remember, what prevents – heals; and what heals – prevents.

SUGAR AND CANCER

Whenever I had visited my friend Dave he was sucking on a soda pop. I would ask, "Dave, what are you doing?" He would reply that the Doc said it was O.K. and that he was cleared to eat and drink anything he wanted. Well-worn advice from the medical professional who probably didn't even have one hour in med school about the fundamentals of nutrition. My answer to that was "Well, sure, if you want to feed the cancer and keep it going and growing!"

NO! STOP THE SUGAR <u>RIGHT NOW!!</u> Do not pass "Go," do not collect $200. Stop right now. Put down that can of pop – I don't care if it's regular or diet. Both are essentially cancer in a can. It's proven that cancer feeds on sugar. It proliferates anaerobically in the cells, destroying the citric acid cycle (Kreb's Cycle), and produces lactic acid as a by-product, which then goes to the liver, is changed back to sugar, then sent back to the cells to feed more cancer. Get the picture? While there is more to it, this is what you need to know. Stop eating anything with sugar or high fructose corn syrup – even honey (sorry) – except in the food supplement known as aloe arborescens (we'll get to that later).

Please understand the facts surrounding this **very serious** matter regarding cancer and sugar – your life may well depend on it. ***Sugar, in virtually any form, effectively (and very quickly) suppresses or disables the human immune system for up to four hours!*** Let's say that another way for a little different perspective. The amount of sugar in a 12-ounce can of soda pop will put your body's only line of defense – the immune system, the single thing in the entire world that can heal your cancer – on its lips for up to four hours. Got it now? If you are a cancer patient, you simply cannot afford it.

And think about this for a moment: If that single "sugar-laced" serving can put the proverbial kibosh on your body's critical cancer-fighting mechanism for up to one-sixth of an entire day, carefully consider the consequences of a daily lifestyle of this standard American diet (yes, the acronym is S.A.D.). It's simply no wonder we're dying of cancer at the rate we are.

Eat no sugar period; no artificial sugar or sweeteners – they *cause* cancer. Only consume stevia or Lo Han (Luo Han Guo – a natural Chinese plant product) if you need a sugar substitute, and get these at your local health food store or co-op in their natural, organic form – not as a mixture or concoction at the grocery store. Better still, use the product Just Like Sugar® that is composed of chicory root, calcium, vitamin C, and the peel of the orange. It is 96% dietary fiber with no calories or sugar. You can't go wrong with this sweet substitute. You can find it at www.justlikesugarinc.com or at Whole Foods.

DAIRY PRODUCTS AND MEAT

If I had cancer, I would not eat any meat or consume any dairy products except organic cottage cheese as part of the Budwig protocol (Chapter

Four). Read the best book every written on the link between diet and cancer (and all disease) by T. Colin Campbell, *The China Study*, and you will know why. Dairy products take a long time to digest and are very acid forming (remember you need to be alkaline). Get your calcium from fruits, vegetables, nuts and seeds, not dairy.

David Gutierrez, a staff writer for *NaturalNews.com*, has some insightful and factual information for you about milk. Please listen closely to the following:

"'From Winston Churchill's wartime order to keep the milk flowing, which was formalized under the 1946 School Milk Act…the idea that it is natural, healthy and an essential part of a good diet has been unchallenged,' writes Andrew Marszal in *The Telegraph*.

"That consensus is wavering. Recently, junior health minister Anne Milton suggested that the national program to provide free milk for children under five should be abolished. And research continues to emerge that milk is neither an essential nor healthy part of the human diet. As Marszal notes, milk contains no nutrient that cannot be found in a balanced, dairy-free diet. Although milk is high in calcium, most of this nutrient cannot actually be absorbed by the human body, making green leafy vegetables a much more effective source. Cow milk, designed for calves, also contains more fat and protein than the human body needs – which is unsur-prising considering that while it takes a human infant 180 days to double its birth weight, it takes a newborn cow only 47 days.

"Much of the concern over milk comes from the hormones and antibiotics inserted into it by modern factory farming. In the book *Alternative Cures*, author Bill Gottlieb quotes cancer specialist Elizabeth Ann Lowenthal as saying, 'All dairy products, even those such as fat-free milk, contain potential tumor-promoting growth hormones that are fed to cows to improve their milk production.'"

O.K. I'm done with milk – and you should be, too. Actually, I have not had a glass of milk in decades. I know that Americans don't want this to be true – this idea that milk is really not good for us. We love our milk and all the products derived from it. From sour cream to cheddar cheese, whipping cream to ice cream, and yogurt to milkshakes – we just don't ever want to give them up. Now that you know the real truth about milk, what will you do? If I were you, I would get my calcium from those "green, leafy vegetables" – not dairy. Once again, it's up to you.

Meat products also take a substantial amount of time to move through the digestive system (pork doesn't even leave the *stomach* for about four and a half hours). Many meats contain toxins as a result of what the animals have been fed and/or what they may have been injected with to super-size them and, in dairy cows, increase the volume of milk produced. Meat digestion requires a lot of energy, producing oxidation and free radicals. A partial result of meat digestion (or lack thereof) is purines – rotten and toxic leftovers – which produce more free radicals (read acid, not good for you). Think about this before scarfing down your next steak. Also, consider that fruits and vegetables transit the entire body within about 18 hours, normally. Meats could take 72 hours or longer and some of it could end up as undigested plaque lining the interior walls of your colon – essentially blocking the absorption of nutrients. While this is not a good scenario for anyone, cancer patients simply cannot afford it.

If a cancer patient absolutely cannot get by without meat (I realize that some won't give it up no matter what), I would suggest small amounts of fresh, coldwater salmon, tuna, halibut, or mackerel – or small portions of free-range/organic chicken or turkey.

STOP EATING THESE

On the "not approved" list are all packaged foods, trans fats, hydrogenated oils (only extra virgin olive oil and coconut oil are allowed), black pepper (very acidic), table salt, junk food (did I even have to mention it?), peanuts, cashews, corn (fungus, aflatoxins), coffee, refined foods, products with yeast (including breads), eggs (unless pregnant – you, not the chicken), alcohol, soy foods (unless fermented or in Reliv™ products), white rice, white potatoes, fruits (except fresh lemons, limes or avocados) – these are no-no's if you have cancer and you must stop eating them now. There will be more on the proper cancer diet in the next chapter. Also, do no cooking with aluminum or chemically coated pots and pans – use glass, ceramic, or specially made stainless steel cookware instead.

TAP WATER, FLUORIDE, CHLORINE

I would never drink regular tap water unless it was an emergency. The story about municipal water systems and the poisons that inhabit them would require an entire book to explain and document. The evidence of tap water toxicity is overwhelming and readily available for your perusal on the Internet. Go see for yourself. The cancer risk among those drinking chlorinated water is 93% higher than those who do not (see quote below).

Most tap water also contains fluoride. Fluoride is a by-product of the aluminum industry, is a deadly poison, and is added to our water systems because of a decade's-old, "fabricated" report stating that it was good for the developing teeth of children. Totally false. Research it yourself – you'll find the truth. No, fluoride is poison – make no mistake. Listen to the following from Gary Null, Ph.D., in his report entitled *The Fluoridation Fiasco – Poison in Your Water*, from the website of Jeff Rense at www.rense. com/health/fluoride1.htm:

"For decades, we have been told a lie, a lie that has led to the deaths of hundreds of thousands of Americans and the weakening of the immune systems of tens of millions more. This lie is called fluoridation. A process we were led to believe was a safe and effective method of protecting teeth from decay is, in fact, a fraud. In recent years it's been shown that fluoridation is neither essential for good health nor protective of teeth. What it does is poison the body. We should all, at this point, be asking how and why public health policy and the American media continue to live with and perpetuate this scientific sham."

Click on that web address above and read the whole story. For additional data on this very controversial subject and the revelation of the truth about fluoride, also see the following sites:

www.holisticmed.com/fluoride

www.just-think-it.com/no-f.htm

This deadly toxin is also added to most toothpaste in the form of sodium monofluorophosphate, or just plain sodium fluoride. Read the back of the tube. It instructs you to contact a doctor or "poison control center" if swallowed. Friends, why would you use this – cancer or not? And why would you let your children use it? Find a toothpaste that has no fluoride. I use "Tom's of Maine" (the no fluoride kind) and alternate that with non-aluminumized baking soda (Bob's Red Mill). Or try Tooth Soap®, made with organic, extra-virgin olive oil, coconut oil, distilled water, and pure essential oils. Yes, it's a little more expensive than your ordinary, poisonous toothpaste at $29.95 for a 6-8 week supply – but well worth it. Find this product at www.toothsoap.com.

Christopher Bryson has written what I consider to be one of the most revealing exposés on fluoride and its history in America that has ever been done. In *The Fluoride Deception*, he pulls no punches, offers no apologies, and presents just the facts, supported by reams and reams of documentation. My interpretation of his work is that fluoride is so incredibly dangerous to the human body and its longevity that it should be banned from any human contact.

The research supporting his claims is overwhelming and entirely indisputable. And yet – and still – fluoride is being added to the toothpaste that our children (and most adults) ingest twice a day and to most of the water that comes out of taps in America's households. Tell me, how is this possible?

You must listen to a few paragraphs of what Chris documents regarding this deadly poison:

"Next time you confront yourself in the bathroom mirror, mouth full of foam, take another look at the toothpaste tube. Most of us associate fluoride with the humdrum issue of better teeth and the promised fewer visits to the dentist. Yet the story of how fluoride was added to our toothpaste and drinking water is an extraordinary, almost fantastic tale. The plot includes some of the most spectacular events in human affairs – the explosion of the Hiroshima atomic bomb, for example. Many of the principal characters are larger than life, such as the 'father of public relations,' Edward L. Bernays, Sigmund Freud's nephew, who was, until now, more famous for his scheme to persuade women to smoke cigarettes. And the twists and turns of the fluoride story are propelled by nothing less than the often grim requirements of accumulating power in the industrial era – the same raw power that is at the beating heart of the American Century.

"Fluoride lies at the elemental core of some of the greatest fortunes that the world has ever seen, the almost unimaginable wealth of the Mellons of Pittsburgh and the DuPonts of Delaware. And no wonder the warning on the toothpaste tube is so dramatic. The same potent chemical that is used to enrich uranium for nuclear weapons, to prepare Sarin nerve gas, and to wrestle molten steel and aluminum from the earth's ore is what we give to our children first thing in the morning and last thing at night, flavored with peppermint, strawberry, or bubble gum.

"Fluoride is so muscular a chemical that it has become a lifeblood of modern industry, pumped hotly each day through innumerable factories, refineries, and mills. Fluoride is used to produce high-octane gasoline; to smelt such key metals as aluminum, steel, and beryllium; to enrich uranium; to make computer circuit boards, pesticides, ski wax, refrigerant gases, teflon, carpets, water-proof clothing, etched glass, bricks and ceramics, and numerous drugs, such as Prozac and Cipro.

"Fluoride's use in dentistry is a sideshow by comparison. But its use in dentistry helps industry, too. How does it work? Call it elemental public relations. Fluoride is so potent a chemical that it's also a grave environmental hazard and a potential workplace poison. So, the industry-sponsored scientists, who first promoted fluoride's use in dentistry, linking the chemical to better teeth and stoutly insisting that, in low doses, it had no other health effect, helped to change fluoride's image from poison to panacea, deflecting attention from the injury that factory fluoride pollution has long wreaked on workers, citizens, and nature."

I know – you had no idea. Not many of us do when it comes to poisons like fluoride because we staunchly believe that our government would not deceive us by burying the truth in layers of lies. Fortunately, when you remove the top layer – that very thick layer that is hard to lift and wants to slap right back down on top of you, that enormous layer that is steeped in deception and fraud – you uncover, to your wonderment, the inner layer of truth that both puzzles and surprises you because it is fresh, smells good, and looks right. Pursue that "inner layer" whether its concerning fluoride or some other idea or substance that stinks to high Heaven.

In Mr. Bryson's pursuit of the truth, he discovered how this industrial poison (fluoride) really and truly afflicts the common man and woman (you and me), and gives a prime example in the next paragraph:

"Thousands of men and women are stalked by fluoride in the modern workplace yet blinkered to its toxic potential, according to Mullenix. In 1998, she met former aluminum workers from Washington State whose health had been ruined by fluoride. 'These men are between thirty and fifty years old and have replaced knees and shoulders; they have leukemias, thyroid problems, and soft tissue diseases. I've never seen such a bunch of young, pathetic people with such health problems. I just don't see the outrage. They are just putting them out as old men, and bringing in younger men, over and over again,' she said."

Are you beginning to get the picture here? Continuous fluoride contact and consumption equates to sickness, disease, and death. It then just remains a question of how fast the reaper arrives.

Simply put, I would not drink chlorinated, fluoridated tap water *ever* – and neither should you. At this time in history, when other mechanisms are available to treat our water effectively, safely, and more economically (ozone, hydrogen peroxide, sodium chlorite, and others), it's truly amazing that our government chooses poisonous substances instead. Please chew on and digest this next statement that comes to us from the following great website, www.healthynewage.com/chlorine-cancer.htm:

"We don't use chlorine because it's the safest or even the most effective means of disinfection; we use it because it's the cheapest. In spite of all our technological advances, we essentially still pour bleach in our water before we drink it. The long-term effects of chlorinated drinking water have just recently been recognized. According to the U.S. Council of Environmental Quality, '*Cancer risk among people drinking chlorinated water is 93% higher than among those whose water does not contain chlorine.'"*

Along these same lines – and regarding something that we just don't think about – is that most of us like to take hot showers, especially in the winter. Unfortunately, we fail to realize that the toxic chlorine is absorbed through our skin and, even more importantly, into our lungs. When the steam from the hot water is inhaled, it goes directly to the lungs which have abundant blood vessels. The chlorine in the steam is immediately absorbed into the blood stream and spread throughout the body. The result? You have just poisoned yourself – and most people innocently poison themselves in this fashion every day. The solution is a $30-$50 filtered showerhead that will eliminate the chlorine. These are available at most hardware or Big Box Stores. Whether I had cancer or not, I would get and install one of these.

ASPARTAME/NUTRASWEET™

If I were to sit down with you for an hour or so and tell you the story of aspartame, a.k.a. Nutrasweet™, when we were finished you would be sitting there with an astonished look on your face and your mouth hanging open. Then you would probably call me a liar because what I had just told you – you would surmise   couldn't possibly be true. Unfortunately, regarding this subject, you would be wrong.

The history of this artificial sweetener is pockmarked with lies and deceit and its mere existence today (and survival) has been accomplished through political chicanery and studies that have been built upon a "foundation of sand." Almost all clinical studies and research on this product reveal, with a rather spectacular certainty, that it causes cancer. In addition, these same studies and other research show that aspartame can increase obesity and is the probable cause of the metabolic syndrome that affects 48 million Americans.

Dr. Russell Blaylock, author of *Excitotoxins: The Taste That Kills*, says it accurately, succinctly, and clearly:

"There is no reason to ever consume this product."

And yet – there it is – in almost every "artificially sweetened" product (we can't call them foods) that we consume. From diet sodas to cereals, jams and jellies to candy and iced tea, juice blends to yogurts, everywhere we look, everywhere we go – it's there – smacking us in the face with its sweetness and promise of no calories. We should be so lucky just to get a punch in the mouth. Instead, what we really receive from this poison that masquerades as a "healthy alternative to sugar," is cancer, obesity, disease, and death.

When aspartame enters the human body it breaks down into fumaric acid (the sting of the fire ant), DKP (think brain cancer), and formaldehyde. See, we are already being embalmed *before* we're dead! Most people know that these things are not good for them. I hope that you do now, too. At about 85-86 degrees, aspartame begins to become unstable and separates into the above identified poisons, uh, excuse me, components. Think for a moment about all that diet pop sitting in the desert during the Gulf War. There are many that relate "Gulf War Syndrome" to this "hot" diet pop.

Dr. Blaylock continues with this:

"The new study released in the *European Journal of Oncology* by Morando Soffritti and co-workers should terrify mothers and all those consuming aspartame-sweetened products. This was a carefully done study which clearly demonstrated a statistically significant increase in several types of lymphomas and leukemias in rats. Both of these malignancies have increased significantly in this country since the widespread use of aspartame."

Geez.

Aspartame is an "excitotoxin" – meaning that it stimulates or excites neural cells ***to death***.

Want more? Sure you do.

My friend, Dr. Betty Martini, is the founder of the worldwide volunteer force, Mission Possible World Health International, which is committed to removing aspartame from our food supply (and, hopefully, from the face of the earth). She has an honorary Doctor of Humanities degree for the work she has done. With 22 years of experience in the medical field, Dr. Martini is uniquely qualified to research and write about aspartame.

Betty is known throughout the world for her work involving aspartame and its deadly effects – especially regarding our children. She's been a featured guest on over 500 talk shows and she appears constantly in magazines and print media. The 1,038 page *Aspartame Disease, An Ignored Epidemic*, by Dr. H.J. Roberts, is dedicated to Dr. Martini. She's made two tours of the United Kingdom, addressed the European Union and, in 2007, made an invited 3-week tour of New Zealand. Betty has made a huge difference, as witnessed by the folding of Europe's largest aspartame producer in 2006, and in forty-seven members of Parliament having signed a bill to ban it from England.

Now that you know Betty, listen closely to what she has to say about aspartame:

"Understand that aspartame starts poisoning when you put it in your mouth. The aspartame industry tries to tell you that aspartate and phenylalanine are some of the building blocks of protein. Dr. Madelon Price, who worked side by side with Dr. John Olney – who tried to prevent approval of aspartame, once explained this very well. She said, the difference is that in food they are bound into complex proteins and linked to complex carbohydrates that take many hours to gradually break down and be slowly absorbed in appropriate quantities into the body by mechanisms destined to do just that. The trouble with aspartame is that, in the acidic warm environment of the stomach, it is broken down very quickly and overwhelms the protective mechanisms that keep aspartate, phenylalanine, and methanol from being taken up by the blood stream too quickly or that dispose of toxic by-products.

"Aspartame, of course, is not an additive but an addictive, excito-neurotoxic, genetically engineered, carcinogenic drug and adjuvant that damages the mitochondria or powerhouse of the cell – and interacts with drugs and vaccines."

The literature and documentation proving the detrimental and carcinogenic effects of aspartame would literally fill your hard drive. In the final analysis, know, beyond any doubt or argument, that this stuff is bad for you. If you want to court Alzheimer's, Lupus, MS, or brain cancer, drink lots of diet soda and have no regard for sugar substitutes – including, and especially, aspartame. If not, avoid it like death itself.

Thanks, Betty. Please keep up the great work.

Soon, if not already, Dr. Martini will be battling *Neotame*, another poison being brought to us by the same folks who gave us aspartame. According to Barbara Peterson (on the www.farmwars.info website), Neotame is a new and improved version of the neurotoxin, aspartame. Barbara gives us some more detail in the following:

"Neotame has similar structure to aspartame – except that, from its structure, it appears to be even more toxic than aspartame. This potential increase in toxicity will make up for the fact that less will be used in diet drinks. Like aspartame, some of the concerns include gradual neurotoxic and immunotoxic damage from the combination of the formaldehyde metabolite (which is toxic at extremely low doses) and the excitotoxic amino acid.

"But surely, this product would be labeled! NOT SO!!! For this little gem, no labeling is required. And it is even included in USDA Certified Organic food. The food labeling requirements for aspartame have now been dropped for Neotame, and no one is clear why this was allowed to happen. Neotame has been ruled acceptable and does not need to be included on the list of ingredients for USDA Certified Organic food items or Certified Kosher products with the official letter "k" inside the circle on labels."

Can you believe it? This, folks, is your FDA at work.

A final note on this subject. The main producer of aspartame, Ajinomoto, has now changed the name of its product to "Aminosweet" and is marketing it as a "natural sweetener." Caveat Emptor (let the buyer beware).

MAMMOGRAMS – SCREENING TESTS – WOMEN'S ISSUES

While I cannot and would not tell women to stop having traditional mammograms, if I were a woman, *I would never have one*. Why? Simply because they are inherently unreliable and, more importantly, they **cause** cancer. Conventional, breast-squishing mammography utilizes ionizing radiation to create an image. And we've already talked about radiation. According to Dr. John W. Goffman, professor emeritus of Cell Biology at the University of California – Berkeley, from his 1995 book, *Preventing Breast Cancer,* page 303, "Our current estimate is that about three-quarters of the current annual incidence of breast cancer in the U.S. is being caused by earlier ionizing radiation, primarily from medical sources. An estimated 75% of recent and current breast cancer cases would not have occurred as they did, in the absence of earlier medical irradiation." I hate to say it but – it's about money, folks.

The website AlternativeMedicine.com states the following:

"As Alternative Medicine has maintained for years, mammograms do far more harm than good. Their ionizing radiation mutates cells, and the mechanical pressure can spread cells that are already malignant (as can biopsies)."

"For years, breast cancer awareness campaigns have urged women over 40 to get a yearly mammogram. When women hesitate to comply, it's often to avoid the discomfort of having their breasts squeezed or the fear of getting called back for more tests, even if it turns out there's no cancer," states Christie Aschwanden in the August 17th edition of the *Los Angeles Times*.

"But screening poses another downside: A routine mammogram can find cancers that would never have become life-threatening, subjecting women to painful and toxic treatments they never actually needed," she continues. And many believe that a majority of these so-called "discovered cancers" were not – and are not – cancers at all.

Here's the clincher from Ms. Aschwanden: "Autopsy studies have found undetected breast cancer in about 37% of women who died of some other cause. And a study of 42,238 Norwegian women published in November (2008) calculated that 22% of symptom-free cancers found on a screening mammogram naturally regressed on their own. The problem is that, even under a microscope, it's impossible to distinguish these different types of cancer from one another, and mammograms are **better at catching the less dangerous kinds"** (emphasis mine).

Ladies, the documented proof is that mammograms and biopsies cause and spread cancer. Do not entertain (I would not) having another unless it is Digital Infrared Imaging (Thermography). The other procedures for screening, i.e., mammography, CT, ultrasound, PET scans, and MRI, only have the ability to detect a tumor once it has reached a certain size – and that is usually *years* after it began to form. On the other hand, thermography, which has been around and FDA approved for 28 years, can detect growths or "malignant cell colonies" up to 10 years in advance of conventional methods (from the *Healing Cancer Naturally* Website). Thermography has the ability to detect the "heat" from tumor or cell capillaries and their secretions and is much more accurate than standard tests. The additional upside? They are a painless, non-contact, and non-invasive testing procedure.

And while we're at it, I would stay away from CT (computed tomography) scans unless absolutely critical (rare). This test is also known as a CAT scan (computerized axial tomography) and literally fills your body with radiation. It was estimated that in 2007 over 62 million CT scans were done – over 4 million on children. And just what did these produce? Over 29,000 new cases of cancer (15,000 fatal) and a whole lot of dollars for the medical industry, according to a study led by Amy Berrington Gonzalez of the National Cancer Institute and published in the *Archives of Internal Medicine*. Again, it's about the money, folks. I have reviewed many sources and the cost of a CT scan can run as low as about $700 or as high as $6,500. The average seems to be somewhere between $2,000-$3,000. Here's what you really need to know. According to Dr. Rebecca Smith-Bindman, as quoted by Richard Knox in his December 15, 2009 article entitled "Radiation From CT Scans May Raise Cancer Risk", from the www.npr.org website, "A single CT scan delivers about the same radiation dose that survivors of the atomic blasts at Nagasaki and Hiroshima endured."

My Dad underwent one atomic bomb after another before he died. If at all possible, stay away from these things. I would. Opt for thermography, MRI's or ultrasound, if you can.

Women of America, please pay especially close attention to this next subject. Another dose of reality hits home when discussing the wearing of bras and this activity's inherent relationship to breast cancer. As always – in this writing – it's time to know the truth instead of what is convenient or politically (or socially) correct. What you are about to hear may cause you great pause – and it should. And to those who have no knowledge of the following, you must ask yourself why you have not been told.

Researchers, Sydney Singer and his wife Soma Grismaijer, did a massive and comprehensive study involving whether bra wearing was, in any way, connected to cancer. What they discovered was startling. Their findings clearly demonstrated that the odds of getting breast cancer dramatically increased with bra-wearing exceeding twelve hours per day. And here's the basic statistical breakdown:

- Women who wore their bras 24 hours per day (really?) had a 3 out of 4 chance of developing breast cancer.
- Women who wore bras more than 12 hours per day – but not to bed – had a 1 out of 7 risk.
- Women who wore their bras less than 12 hours per day had a 1 out of 152 risk (are you getting this?).
- Women who wore bras rarely or never, had a 1 out of 168 chance of developing breast cancer.

The overall correlation between 24-hour bra wearing and not wearing one at all was calculated to be a 125-fold difference! So what's the deal, you ask?

Dr. Ralph L. Reed, Ph.D., says it this way – and he's *spot on*:

"Lymphatic circulation in many tissues (especially the primary lymphatics) is highly dependent on MOVEMENT. When you sit for a long time on an airplane flight, your feet and ankles can swell because lymphatic circulation goes to near zero. Wearing a bra, especially a constricting one with underwires, and especially to bed, prevents normal lymphatic flow and would likely lead to anoxia (lower than normal oxygen content), which has been related to fibrosis – which has been linked to increased cancer risk. Every subtle bounce of the breast while moving, walking, running, etc., gently massages the breast and increases the lymphatic flow and thus cleans the breast of toxins and wastes that arise from cellular metabolism."

From the "007b.com" website we hear it said in another way:

"The main reason why tight bras are bad for breast health is because they restrict the lymph flow in your breasts. There are numerous lymph pathways and lymph nodes in the armpits, under the breasts, and in-between the breasts. Normally, the lymph fluid washes out waste materials and other toxins away from the breasts, but bras (and especially push-up bras) inhibit this action, so toxins can start to accumulate in the breast, and that can help cancer to develop. In other words, bras inhibit the way our bodies normally cleanse themselves and get rid of cancer cells and toxins like PCBs, DDT, dioxin, benzene and other carcinogenic chemicals that cling to the body's fatty tissues – like the breast. In fact, if you find a lump in your breast, it may very well be filled with lymph fluid that was not able to move away from the breast tissue.

"Bra-wearing may also be connected to cancer in other ways. Wearing bras slightly increases the temperature of the breast tissue, and women who wear bras have higher levels of the hormone prolactin. Both of these may influence breast cancer formation."

Women of America, the evidence is in and it appears to be very conclusive. Consider doing what is right for your breast health – not just what looks best, is more fashionable, or convenient. At a minimum, take that "double-barreled sling shot" off when you are at home and/or in a private setting – and consider "something" not quite as restricting. You may be very happy that you did.

Another very important application to potential breast cancer inception involves the use of common, off-the-store-shelf, deodorants and anti-perspirants. While this subject is important to both women and men, women, it appears, run the greater risk.

A study done by P.D. Darbre at the University of Reading in the United Kingdom, and reported in the *Journal of Inorganic Biochemistry*, September 2005 issue, states the following:

> "Aluminum salts are used as the active antiperspirant agent in underarm cosmetics, but the effects of widespread, long-term and increasing use remain unknown, especially in relation to the breast, which is a local area of application. Clinical studies showing a disproportionately high incidence of breast cancer in the upper outer quadrant of the breast, together with reports of genomic instability in outer quadrants of the breast, provide supporting evidence for a role for locally applied cosmetic chemicals in the development of breast cancer. Aluminum is known to have a genotoxic profile capable of causing both DNA alterations and epigenetic effects, and this would be consistent with a potential role in breast cancer if such effects occurred in breast cells. Given the wide exposure of the human population to antiperspirants, it will be important to establish dermal absorption in the local area of the breast and whether long-term low level absorption could play a role in the increasing incidence of breast cancer."

Well, yeah, I would say that would be pretty important. And here's the real pertinent relevance to women. The majority of women in America (and now many other countries) shave their underarms routinely. As a result, the deodorants and antiperspirants have direct contact with the skin and are absorbed readily. Conversely, most men (and some women) who do not shave their underarms – and, because of the hair growth in that region – have less direct skin contact with these "cosmetics."

It should be well known (but isn't) that we were meant to perspire as a way to rid the body of toxins and as a method to cool the body. Now, add this up. When we load our underarms with a thick, carcinogenic paste, liquid, or spray, we not only don't perspire there but we absorb more toxins. Just how much sense does this make? I believe you get the point.

Whenever possible, utilize natural "deodorants" (there are many) and avoid chemical-laced antiperspirants. You can even make your own – there are several recipes involving corn starch, baking soda, essential oils, witch hazel, etc. Cruise the Internet and find what suits you.

WARNING – The following may shock you (and it should) and you probably will find it hard to believe. You simply will not be able to accept that it is true. I assure you – it is. You have been warned:

> "'Anaphylactic shock,' 'foaming at mouth,' 'grand mal convulsion,' 'coma,' and 'now paralyzed' are just a few of the startling descriptions included in a new federal report describing the complications from Merck & Co.'s Gardasil medication for sexually transmitted human papillomavirus – which has been proposed as mandatory for all schoolgirls."

This headline paragraph led off an entire article in the *WorldNetDaily* in its Tuesday, November 16th, 2010, edition entitled "Death Toll Linked to Gardasil Vaccine Rises." I warned you that it would be unbelievable. And while I'm not going to include the entire news story here, you need to know a little more. Hang on to something:

> "The document (mentioned above) was obtained from the U.S. Food and Drug Administration by *Judicial Watch*, a Washington group that investigates and prosecutes government corruption, and it has details of 10 deaths just since September."

And don't for a second believe that the FDA gave up this document easily. It continues:

> "'Given all the questions about Gardasil, the best public health policy would be to re-evaluate its safety and to prohibit its distribution to minors. In the least, governments should rethink any efforts

to mandate or promote this vaccine for children,' said *Judicial Watch* President, Tom Fitton. The organization's work uncovered reports of about one death each month since last fall, bringing the total death toll from the drug to at least 18 and as many as 20. There also were 140 'serious' reports of complications including about three dozen classified as life-threatening, 10 spontaneous abortions, and a half a dozen cases of Guillain-Barre Syndrome."

And now they want to prescribe this for young boys, too? Are you kidding me? While the drug companies may consider the deaths and complications as acceptable collateral damage, I do not – and no one of good conscience should. Listen to Barbara Hollingsworth in the March 30th, 2010, *Washington Examiner*:

"As of January 31, 2010, forty-nine unexplained deaths following Gardasil injections have been reported to the Centers for Disease Control and Prevention's Vaccine Adverse Event Reporting System. By contrast, 52 deaths are attributed to unintended acceleration in Toyotas, which triggered a $2 billion recall. No recall for Gardasil, which is required for sixth grade girls in D.C., Maryland, Virginia, and many other states."

Friends, it's "High Noon" and time to recall this drug that is taking the lives of our teenage daughters. As a matter of fact, we've gone far beyond the time to question every drug and every vaccine that the government, FDA, and pharmaceutical companies try to foist upon the most defenseless, innocent, and precious of all – our children. As a preventative for cervical cancer – Gardasil is a joke, and a very bad and sad one. There are many other non-toxic ways to prevent cervical cancer – and all cancers. They're in this book. Keep reading.

MEN'S ISSUES

Gentlemen, I'll keep this brief, succinct, and very understandable – for you just can't make a mistake with this.

In most cases – and for most men diagnosed with prostate cancer – this "non-disease" **will not kill you!** I hope you get this message and will pass it along. Many of us have not and the "prostatectomy line" isn't getting any shorter. Haven't we heard the news? If not, listen up and I'll give you the latest on this.

The founder of the PSA (prostate specific antigen) test that measures a protein released by prostate cells that "supposedly" indicates that cancer **might** be present, has **recanted**. Let's hear it straight from the horse's mouth. Here's Dr. Thomas Stamey, M.D., professor of urology and lead author of the study that was recently published in the *Journal of Urology* regarding prostate tissues removed and examined over 20 years:

> "The PSA era is over in the United States. Our study raises a very serious question of whether a man should even use the PSA test for prostate cancer screening any more.

> "Our job now is to stop removing every man's prostate who has prostate cancer," said Stamey. "We originally thought we were doing the right thing, but we are now figuring out how we went wrong. Some men need prostate treatment but certainly not all of them."

I say "good on ya" Doc. Being willing to step up and admit a critical mistake that has costs tens of thousands of men their prostates (and more), is a great start. It's no consolation, however, to those who have been maimed, disfigured, made dysfunctional, and worse. And, unfortunately, many guys – and many surgeons – haven't gotten the word on this.

Men, stay away from any medical advice regarding immediate prostate removal or practitioner who says that "we need to do surgery right away." And talk to someone who has already had the procedure done – if he has survived. In most instances, he will tell you a very frightening tale about the nightmare that was created when he submitted to the knife. Stories of permanent incontinence, urological problems, and erectile dysfunction are common. It's a continuing litany of tragedy that envelops and smothers the simple fact that men with prostate cancer who do absolutely nothing – having no conventional, allopathic intervention at all – live just as long or longer than those who choose mainstream intervention. And they also have a far better quality of life. I'm not suggesting, however, that men with cancer do nothing.

You see, guys, if we live long enough, most of us will get prostate cancer – to one degree or another. If we live to be 100 and die of "old age," at autopsy the good doctor will probably discover that we had prostate cancer.

Dr. Stamey concludes with this:

"What we didn't know in the early years is that benign growth of the prostate is the most common cause of a PSA level between 1 and 10."

While on rare occasions surgery may indeed be necessary to save the life of a man with severe prostate cancer (that is, he will be dead in the next 48 hours or so without it), men should do their homework on this and understand that surgery is definitely not the first thing and should be an absolute last resort. Only about 226 out of 100,000 men over the age of 65 die of prostate cancer – a rate of .003 percent. Guys, you're much more likely to die of something else – like getting struck by lightning. Think about it.

SUNLIGHT – VITAMIN D

Contrary to popular belief, the sun is your friend, not your enemy. Now listen closely because there's going to be a quiz later. I am about to tell you a few things that you will seriously question because you have been conditioned by the mainstream media and advertisers to believe otherwise. Pay close attention to the following one-liners:

The incidence of skin cancer (including melanoma) is highest in those parts of the world where sunscreen use is highest.

Melanoma is more common in people who work indoors than outdoors and often forms on parts of the body that get the least sun exposure.

And last, but certainly not least, most sunscreens contain carcinogenic substances.

Yes, you heard it right.

Vitamin D is one of the most critical and important nutrients for cancer patients (and virtually everyone else) – so important that I struggled with not writing a whole chapter on it.

Almost all of us are deficient in vitamin D3 – period. While studies show that 70% of whites and 97% of African Americans are deficient, I suspect the rates are actually higher (than 70%) with lighter skinned folks. Those with dark skin pigmentation block the needed ultraviolet light that is necessary for their skin to produce the vitamin D.

Recently, our vitamin-resistant governmental agencies very reluctantly raised the almost negligible RDA of 200 IU (international units) to 600 IU for this vitamin. You would have thought that someone had a gun to their heads – it was obviously excruciatingly painful for them. After all, this is a natural product – not a drug. How can it possibly be useful? Well, I've got news for you. Six hundred international units is still woefully low. And here's proof.

Caucasian skin produces about 10,000 IU of vitamin D with a scant 20-30 minutes of direct summer sun exposure. I know people who are out in the sun almost all summer long – and the rest of the year, too. They have no skin cancer, do not use sunscreens (that cause cancer), and are some of the healthiest people I know.

The pure and simple fact is that vitamin D (specifically, D3) *prevents 77% of all cancers!* Did you get that? A study conducted by Creighton University School of Medicine that involved almost 1,800 women in good health proved that supplementation of calcium and vitamin D reduced cancer rates by this amazing 77% (as reported in the *American Journal of Clinical Nutrition*). The intake of vitamin D in the control group of this study was only 1,100 IU daily. Imagine what might have occurred if they were given 4,000-5,000 IU daily!

You need vitamin D, especially vitamin D3 (cholecalciferol) to help process calcium and phosphorus and recent studies show that this substance, processed in the liver and kidneys, promotes the death of cancer cells. The problem is that the good food sources of vitamin D are not (for the most part) on the cancer diet: beef liver, salmon, mackerel, sardines, and egg yolks. So where do you get it? From the two best sources; the sun and cod liver oil.

Find a good cod liver oil, however. Most companies, believe it or not, are taking the natural vitamin D out and replacing it with a synthetic form of this vitamin (which then ceases to be a real vitamin at all). I take Green Pasture's Blue Ice™ Fermented Cod Liver Oil. Use this or study-up and find your own source. Listen to what Dr. Bruce West says about cod liver oil (CLO) in his recent *Health Alert* Newsletter, May 2010, Volume 27, Issue 5:

"If you have had breast cancer, if you are at high risk for breast cancer, if you are afraid of getting breast cancer, or if you are just smart, *you will take cod liver oil* (CLO) for the rest of your life. Aside from being a sacred food and elixir that has profound and wonderful health benefits, CLO and its vitamin D are profoundly linked with breast cancer prevention.

"In fact, one of the world's leading vitamin D researchers, Dr. Cedric Garland, recently told a gathering at the Toronto School of Medicine's 'Diagnosis and Treatment of Vitamin D Deficiency' conference, that breast cancer is a disease so directly related to vitamin D deficiency that a woman's risk of contracting the disease can be 'virtually eradicated' by elevating her vitamin D status to what vitamin D scientists consider to be natural levels.

"As we have stated previously, there are many forms of Vitamin D. And there are still many forms of vitamin D that we simply do not even know about. So it makes sense to raise your levels with the whole food that is super-rich in the whole vitamin D with all its variations. That food is ***Blue Ice ™ Fermented Cod Liver Oil.*** We use it in the form of capsules, with 2-5 capsules daily being the most common dose to bring vitamin D levels back to normal."

With breast cancer – or any type of cancer – use cod liver oil in its purest and most complete form.

And get out into the sun every day, if you can. There's no substitute for good, old-fashioned sunshine. Just don't burn yourself to a crisp – that's actually ***not*** good for you. And in the northern latitudes in the winter, find a tanning bed that is high in UVB rays and use it.

Make note, however, that after a sunlight/UVB session, wait a bit before showering. Danna Norek, a citizen journalist for *NaturalNews.com*, tells us why:

"After UV exposure, your skin produces a powdery substance that is then absorbed into the skin and converted to vitamin D by the body. If you wash this off too early, you interfere with the amount of vitamin D made and, hence, do not get the full benefit."

I would get into the sun for at least 15 minutes every day that I could. And when I could not – or if I lived in a place with little direct sunshine – I would substitute a good vitamin D3 supplement (4,000-5,000 IU minimum) for my lack of rays. Regardless, I would take cod liver oil every day.

Vitamin D and sunlight. These are two very important things I would implement into my life (and I have), even if I didn't have cancer. You should, too.

CARCINOGENIC PRODUCTS

Another thing I would do is to seriously review everything I touch and put on my body each day. This list includes deodorant, shaving cream, cologne, perfume, soap, make-up, lotion, hair spray, dishwashing liquid, etc., etc. The inventory is extensive and these products can contain (and most do) many known carcinogens including acetone, methylene chloride and others. Get these things out of your life. Go to the local co-op or health store – you'll find "natural" replacements for almost all of these.

There are now many, many private and public companies that have gone the *natural* route when it comes to cosmetics, personal care items, lotions and, basically, anything that one would put on their body. Friends, as convenient and cheap as it is to procure our lotions, potions, and magic rejuvenating elixirs from the local supermarket, pharmacy, or big box store, in most cases, it's the wrong thing to do – and here's why:

What you put on your skin will find its way into your bloodstream in **28 seconds!**

I'm sure you had no idea. Do you think we should be a little more careful about these decisions – especially when *known carcinogens* are involved? I do.

Two premier companies that I would recommend (I receive nothing for mentioning them) are Arbonne and Shaklee. As I stated previously, there are many, many others and you should choose who you like after investigating and finding the purest and safest products. Arbonne offers about everything you could need in cosmetics that are Swiss formulated, vegan approved, Kosher, and 100% pure (natural – no toxins). As a sidelight, they also offer vegan protein shakes which are a great source of "non-meat/non-milk" protein for cancer patients.

Shaklee also offers fabulous, non-toxic, natural cosmetics at reasonable prices. I must mention here that I am very enamored with Shaklee's new product called *Vivix®*. This company touts it as the "world's best cellular anti-aging supplement." *Vivex®* is perfectly safe, all natural, and has been shown (in lab studies) to protect and repair cellular DNA. This product also supports immune health. Shaklee states that *Vivex®* has the equivalent amount of resveratrol (think good for you and bad for cancer) found in 3,000 glasses of red wine – of course, without the alcohol! Do yourself a favor and investigate this product and the many testimonies to what it has done for people with severe health challenges – including cancer.

Keep in mind that what both of these companies offer – and all comparable businesses that market similar natural products – will be slightly more expensive than traditional lines that have questionable or carcinogenic ingredients that you can't pronounce. And, through experience, I have discovered they are well worth it.

DETOXIFICATION

After you have stopped doing the things that promote or feed your cancer, you must begin the detoxification process that will eliminate the poisons that have played an integral part in the development of your disease and will feed its growth if allowed to remain in your body. Actually, we should all "detox" on a regular basis.

I would start with a colon cleanse. Many medical professionals (mostly alternative doctors and health practitioners who understand the functions of the human body) believe that most disease begins in the colon. And it makes perfect sense. If this organ is encrusted with plaque, mucous, undigested foods – and who knows what else – this instrument of nutrient absorption and waste elimination will not function properly and will simply become ineffective and, ultimately, diseased. I'm always shocked to learn that many people have a bowel movement only once every few days or so. Now, let's see. Three meals (or more) a day, every day, one bowel movement every few days – hmm…… Where's everything going? Interesting question.

Please carefully consider the following statement: Doesn't it make perfect sense that if you eat three times a day you should have three bowel movements a day? The obvious answer is "of course it does," but, in most people's lives, it simply is not the case. If you are not "going" at least once a day minimum, you're in trouble. The "back-up" will fester, ferment and rot while you complain of bloating, gas, acid reflux, heartburn, cramps, candida, "pot-gut" and every other digestive disturbance known to man. Forgive me, but the fact is that most of us are literally full of crap.

Many years ago, a well-known Hollywood celebrity and actor died and an autopsy was performed. This man was known to have cancer. It was discovered during the post-death examination that he had approximately twenty-five pounds of encrusted fecal matter in his colon! No wonder he had cancer!

Cleanse your colon whether you have cancer or not and drink ionized water (more on this in Chapter Six). There are many different recipes to accomplish this task. Go on line, review the list of protocols, then choose the one that sounds best to you. This site is excellent and I would go here first:

www.the-natural-path.com/toxic-cleansing.html

There's no magic here and you will know if it is working. Utilize a protocol, however, that is natural – no drugs, chemicals, etc. Or go down to your local health or natural food store and ask them what is the best. Don't scrimp on a few dollars here; they are not expensive. Better yet, make an appointment with a local naturopath and get his or her input. This professional will steer you in the right direction. This process is critically important because of two basic things. Firstly, upon completion of this cleanse, you will be much more able to absorb the nutrients and fluids that you will be flooding your body with as part of your new anti-cancer diet and, secondly, your digestive system will now be prepared to eliminate, more efficiently, the debris (once you start to destroy cancer cells) and the waste that naturally flows through it.

Once the colon is cleansed, move immediately to the gall bladder and liver cleanses – utilizing the same process (selection of protocols). Investigate, find the one that will work for you, procure the program, and then proceed expeditiously. These are also referenced and detailed at the website mentioned above and many "recipes" are free. Fresh lemons and a good, organic milk thistle supplement are also excellent for detoxifying and supporting the liver. For now, women with breast cancer avoid the milk thistle.

Lastly, we move on to the "mother of all cleanses", the "parasite purge." I know what you're thinking. Me? Parasites? No way! **_WAY!_** Virtually all humans host at least one – or one type – of parasite. Most of us – many more. And you've got to get them out of your body if you want to heal. The late Hulda Regehr Clark insisted that the cause of all cancers was a single parasite – the human intestinal fluke. She believed that if you kill this parasite, the cancer stops immediately and the tissue becomes normal again. While I'm not sure that I would buy into this theory lock, stock, and barrel,

I do believe (and so should you) that parasites are a problem and we need to get rid of them.

Again, there are many programs available to purge these creepy little creatures from our internal crevices. Personally, I like Dr. Clark's method because it not only targets the parasites, but their eggs, as well (yes, they lay eggs inside you). She suggests that a combination of the tincture of the "green hull" of the Black Walnut, Wormwood (from the Artemisia shrub), and Common Cloves (from the Clove tree) will kill adults and developmental stages of at least 100 parasites (they must be used together). Do a little research, find the cleanse that you feel is best, and go for it. This is what I would do, even if I didn't have cancer.

Cherie Calbom is world-renowned as the "Juice Lady" and has written many books on health and healing. I am honored to call her my friend. Listen to what Cherie has to say about detoxing and its importance in one of her recent works entitled, *The Complete Cancer Cleanse*:

"Detoxification is a normal process of eliminating wastes and toxins from the colon, liver, kidneys, gallbladder, lungs, skin, lymph, and blood. This is one of the body's most basic functions and happens without a thought, like the beating of the heart. However, in our polluted world, the body's systems and organs, which were once functioning in a less-polluted world and capable of clearing out unwanted substances, are now completely overloaded. This means toxins remain in our tissues, clog our organs, poison our blood, and weaken our immune system.

"When immune activity is compromised, immune cells, such as the natural killer cells that are responsible for destroying cancer cells, are unable to do their job properly. A compromised immune system is often a key factor in immune-compromised diseases such as cancer.

"Who should cleanse? The answer is simple! Everybody should cleanse – and especially everyone with cancer."

Cherie continues with what I believe is the most important part of this detoxification protocol. She quotes Anne and David Frahm from their book, *The Cancer Battle Plan*, with the following:

"It seems clear that if a cancer warrior is going to have any hope of ultimately conquering cancer and winning back health, a very aggressive process needs to be undertaken to reverse the chronic degeneration of the body of which cancer is a symptom. It all comes down to changing the body's toxic chemistry through the metabolic processes of detoxification and diet – and the sooner the better."

Folks, that *is* the battle plan. And you'll hear it time and time again from those who know and have proven that detoxification and diet are the keys – and the baseline – to healing cancer. Healed bodies speak the truth about what works, and these two ingredients are well-worn and time-tested.

Get Cherie's book if you can. She is one of the kindest souls you will ever meet – a gentle woman who pours her heart into her work to help people stay healthy and heal when they are not.

If I needed help with a detoxification process or program and could travel, I can tell you exactly where I would go – and that would be We Care Spa™ in Desert Hot Springs, California. Known as the "spa to the stars," this facility is probably the most well known healing and detoxing location in the world. And although it has catered to the Hollywood elite – as well as health conscious people from all over the planet – everyone is welcome and can find respite here.

Offering packages from the "8-day renewal" to the "3-day tune-up," this gorgeous 60-acre compound has been providing cleansing and anti-aging protocols for over 25 years. From colon hydrotherapy to digestive release massage, detox baths, and organic foods, We Care Spa™ virtually has it all. Organic vegetable juices, enzymes, barley grass and wheat grass supplements are just a small sample of what's on the menu – and the anti-cancer diet and protocol features all of these. Specialized equipment, Jacuzzi's, and detoxifying infrared saunas are all available for use.

You'll simply find no better place if you need to detox (mentally and physically) – and learn how to do so in the future. Here you can relax in an environment that is aesthetically pleasing, comfortable, all-inclusive – and private. Many other rejuvenation services and treatments are also available.

One might assume that this kind of place would be very, very expensive. Not so. Actually, it's quite a bargain for what you get. After all, what kind of a price can we put on full body detoxification and restoration (essential for cancer patients) that might just save our lives? I'll leave that one up to you.

Contact the staff at We Care Spa™ through their website and get the full details: www.wecarespa.com.

Another thing to consider is coffee enemas. **WHAT??** You heard that right. And, no, that doesn't include latte's and mochas. As we all know, people don't want to talk about the "e" word (enemas), they don't want to hear about why they are important and what they do, they just want to ignore the subject altogether. These are, however, often a necessary part of a cancer patient's recovery that cannot be ignored or wished-away. And despite what you might be thinking or what you may have heard, there is real science behind this specific procedure and it works efficiently and effectively to help the liver dispose of toxins and debris. We will talk more about this in Chapter Seven – please prepare yourself. While this is a major and ongoing detox protocol required for most cancer sufferers, it is not always critical and mandatory right away – and not absolutely necessary for all patients.

EXERCISE

Statistics show us (no, they really prove) that exercise can ward off disease of all types, especially cancer, while inactivity invites the onset and proliferation of these events.

Simply put, everyone who is able (Dr. approved, of course) should be doing some sort of exercise – sick or not. Lack of physical activity will increase the risk of breast cancer, according to Dr. Elizabeth Smoots. She also states that "a 50 percent decrease in the rate of colon cancer was found in those with the highest levels of physical activity" and that "walking less than 20 minutes a week was associated with twice the risk of pancreatic cancer compared to walking more than four hours a week."

Dr. Smoots goes on to say that "sedentary women had a 72 percent higher rate of melanoma skin cancer than those exercising five to seven days a week. In men, the rate was 56 percent higher." Guess what? Yes, many of these "exercisers" are out in the sun absorbing those UVB rays! There goes the cancer and sunscreen industry's claim that you get melanoma from sun exposure!

You get the picture. I would be willing to bet 4 pieces of red chalk, 3 cat eye marbles, and 2 cents that America could cut its cancer rates in half if we would only exercise. But, I know, we're way too busy for that.

Ladies and gentlemen, boys and girls, and those with cancer who are physically able, get off your tired (and increasingly sick) butts and get moving! Without a doubt, you will be healthier, have more energy, ward off disease of all types, and have a greater capacity to heal sickness throughout your life.

At a minimum and, once again – if they can – cancer patients should start walking and get their blood moving. Get on a mini-trampoline or rebounder and jump or bounce (even lightly) up and down. This exercise is one of the best to help the lymphatic system move the toxins out of the body. And make no mistake; with cancer, you not only need this, it is **required.** If you are unable to do this, find a specialist who does lymphatic massage to help you meet this critical need.

There can be no argument that people who are active and exercise regularly are healthier – and stay that way. They also heal more rapidly.

C'mon – let's get going, America! After all, we really don't have a shortage of doctors in our country, we just have too many sick people. And we don't lack for hospitals, oncologists, radiation equipment or chemotherapy drugs – *we just have way too many cancer patients!*

CANCER TESTING

Earlier in this Chapter I mentioned the "Navarro Urine Test." I believe that this test is probably one of the most accurate detectors of both cancer and *how much* cancer you have. It will also reliably (statistics show 95% or better) predict the presence of this disease up to three years prior to the discovery of lumps, tumors, or blood markers, and is superior to blood tests and other detection methodologies.

The Navarro Urine Test measures HCG (human chorionic gonadotropin). HCG is a glycoprotein hormone and its presence in the urine reflects that the "host" (you) is pregnant, has suffered a serious and traumatic injury, or has cancer. If you can rule out the first two, the third is generally certain. Dr. Manuel Navarro found that this hormone was present and elevated in virtually all types of cancer. We won't get into the details here. Dr. Navarro was no piker. He was an internationally recognized cancer researcher and oncologist with over 100 major scientific papers to his credit. He treated cancer patients for over 25 years with Laetrile – with great success. The late Dr. Navarro was Professor of Medicine and Surgery at the University of Santo Tomas, in Manila, and was also an Associate Member of the National Research Council of the Philippines and a Fellow of the Philippine College of Physicians and the Philippine Society of Endocrinology and Metabolism. He developed his testing procedure in the late 1930's and died in 1994. His son now carries on his work and does the testing of submitted urine samples. You can go to the following website to learn all about the test, how to do it, and where to send it for evaluation:

www.new-cancer-treatments.org/Articles/Determine

Better yet, you can contact my friend, Joe Karlovich, and his crew at the Joe Ball Company. They have developed a kit that will guide you through this process step by step. Each kit contains everything you need to complete and forward the sample and includes beakers, measuring glass, acetone, iso-propanol, filters, etc. Also included are procedures, patient information forms, USPS Express Mail envelopes, pre-addressed labels, and customs declaration forms. They've thought of everything and it's all there.

The kit sells for $39.99 and includes enough materials to run two tests. Reorder kits are only $19.99. International kits are available for $29.99 and are less expensive because they cannot ship the acetone and rubbing alcohol needed for the testing – the recipient has to acquire their own. I highly recommend this kit – and this type of testing. Go to www.joeballcompany. com to order. And if you use the coupon code "AACI" at checkout, you will receive 10% off everything in your cart – compliments of the American Anti-Cancer Institute and the Joe Ball Company.

I have known many who have done it and I have seen the results. This test and process works, is reliable, and is a great way to monitor your progress as you watch your cancer go away. This is what I would do.

ADVOCATES

A cancer diagnosis is devastating – at a minimum. Your entire life – and the sum of its parts – all changes when the "Big C" comes home to roost. Your emotions go into high gear and there is a definite possibility that they will turn you in the wrong direction. We will deal with "emotional detoxification" in Chapter Nine.

What you must do first, though, what you must do right now, is to find an "advocate" – someone who will get onboard this train with you and ride in the seat right next to yours, holding your hand and guiding and supporting you on this journey. Without an advocate, you are traversing the "minefield" of cancer therapies alone. And battling this disease by yourself can be frustrating, irritating, emotionally draining and, as a result, often ends tragically. So find a friend, a family member, a group, anyone who will sign-on to march lock step with you in your quest for healing, until you are well. Do it right away. I would make an "advocate" one of my top priorities.

Always remember, don't panic – you almost always have time. Get your protocol together, do your homework, question all medical advice (question all advice – no matter where it comes from – question my advice, and check it out). Stop doing the things that promote your cancer – start doing the things that will lead you to healing. That's what I would do.

CHAPTER FOUR

"THE CANCER DIET: OXYGEN RICH AND ALKALINE"

"Food as a key to health represents a powerful challenge to conventional medicine, which is fundamentally built on drugs and surgery. The widespread communities of nutrition professionals, researchers and doctors are, as a whole, either unaware of this evidence or reluctant to share it. Because of these failings, Americans are being cheated out of information that could save their lives."

T. Colin Campbell, Ph.D. – *The China Study*

FOOD – it can heal you – and it can kill you. It can be good for what "ails" you or make you sick as a dog. Food can be fried and fricasseed, baked, boiled and butchered. And the list goes on.

The problem today in America – and the rest of the industrialized world – is that we have loaded the basic food groups with artificial sweeteners, trans fats, synthetic additives and preservatives, hormones, dyes – another list that goes on and on.

Folks, do we simply not understand that we weren't meant to eat these things? Whatever happened to fruits and vegetables, seeds and nuts, whole grains, oatmeal – real foods with phytonutrients, vitamins, minerals and protein? And, no, to reiterate a fact from earlier in this writing, French fries are not a vegetable.

The majority of cancer is caused by what we eat and drink! You can dispute that if you like, but the evidence is in and irrefutable, and you simply won't win that argument. I am not intentionally trying to offend anyone when I tell you the following truth: we have arguably become a nation of fat, lazy, unhealthy people. In no uncertain terms, we have literally "super-sized" ourselves. Two-thirds of us are overweight and a full third (or more) are obese. The most unfortunate thing about this behavior is that our kids are growing up just like Mom and Dad. *What has happened to us?* We don't exercise anymore, we sit for hours in front of the T.V. (there's a reason they call it the "boob tube"), we invest weeks of our lives playing video games, consume more booze, coffee, and soda pop than ever, and many still smoke like a chimney. Tell me, what's that all about?

Then, when our bodies begin to fail us, we want to question why we are sick, why we get heart disease, diabetes, arthritis and cancer. Sorry, we can't pretend any longer that there is some cosmic mystery surrounding how this happens. It's time to put down the fork, get our tired rear ends out of the easy chair, and stop this nonsense right now – whether you are sick or not. And if you have cancer, you need to change your lifestyle and your diet *yesterday.* So, let's get started.

ACID – ALKALINE

Most people have "acidosis" as a result of environmental conditions and, largely, because of what they put in their mouths. We eat acidic foods (or acid-forming foods), our bodies become acidic and, as a result, an inner terrain is established that is ripe for every kind of disease, bacteria, fungus, virus and parasite.

I've never known of a cancer patient that was too alkaline. Typically, those with cancer have pH readings in the 4's and 5's (very acidic). Low blood oxygen levels are also characteristic of those with this "disease." Remember that cancer hates – and cannot live in – an alkaline environment.

It also fears and expires when confronted with oxygen. Doesn't it make complete sense then, that to reverse cancer, we must oxygenate and alkalinize our bodies? You would think that this would be the quintessential "no-brainer." Sadly, our doctors pay no attention to this *fact* – and neither do we.

Dr. Gary Tunsky wrote a book entitled *The Battle for Health Is Over pH*. Here's what he says about cancer, acid, oxygen, and pH:

"This acid fermentation process is what we label as cancer. It's my conclusion, based on years of research and study, that cancer is nothing more than an electrical disturbance at the sub-atomic and DNA level caused by oxygen deprivation, dehydration, cellular intoxication, lack of circulation and electrical flow that leads to cell asphyxiation, finally resulting in cell mutation.

"The battle between life and death and humanity's struggle with sickness is over pH. This is not a complicated issue to understand. As long as the body has sufficient alkaline potential from a well-balanced diet and all of its elimination routes are open, cell-damaging acids can be safely neutralized and excreted from the body before cellular damage takes place.

"If we habitually consume fresh, organic, high alkaline forming fruits, vegetables, nuts, seeds and legumes grown in rich topsoil, avoiding as much as humanly possible the 'acid landmines' of our modern civilization, we can properly alkalize the body and stay healthy. When our blood contains living nutrients, our body's cell metabolism and pH are in proper balance. When our cells are properly nourished, hydrated, and oxygenated, it is virtually impossible for us to become unwitting victims of illness and disease."

With cancer, we must do everything possible to strengthen and build the immune system – that is what will ultimately heal us. And this is where the "cancer diet" enters in. Please keep in mind this fact, however – anything that we do or eat that doesn't support this protocol *hurts it*. We must get our pH back up to seven or above, and food (and alkaline water) is the key.

FIRST, DIET TIPS

Prior to outlining the proper cancer diet protocol, here is a list of things that I would do first – or in conjunction with – the new diet regimen:

- Throw away the microwave – it kills the enzymes in food.
- Eat 80% of food raw (if possible). This includes juicing.
- Throw away aluminum cookware and other "coated" cookware and cook exclusively in glass, ceramic, or certified stainless steel pots and pans (checkout Saladmaster® cookware).
- Eat "certified organic" – if it is affordable.
- Don't wash fruits and vegetables in chlorinated water (more on this in Chapter Six).
- No black pepper – it is one of the most acidic foods on the planet.
- No table salt/iodized salt. Eat only quality "full spectrum" salt like "Himalayan" with natural trace minerals (local health food store – more on this later).
- For the very few foods that are cooked using oil, use only extra-virgin olive oil, nut oil(s), or coconut oil.
- No commercial salad dressings – only those made using olive oil, coconut oil, nut oils, oregano oil, lemon, lime, apple cider vinegar, etc. Bragg makes wonderful organic salad dressings and has the premier organic apple cider vinegar.
- Eat virtually nothing that comes in a package, box or can from the local supermarket (eat fresh foods).
- Eat no meat, or very little if you feel you absolutely must to survive. And you won't like this, but eat it as close to raw as you

can. Preferably, ingest only small amounts of fresh cold-water salmon, halibut, tuna, mackerel, or free-range (organically raised) chicken or turkey. A little wild game meat may also be used (key words – " a little"). Steam or cook lightly.

- No milk or milk products, cheese, yogurt, etc., except organic, low-fat cottage cheese in the Budwig Protocol (more on this later). No butter, no margarine.

- No coffee or alcohol. The exceptions are small amounts of coffee made with 9.5 pH water or Ganoderma coffee (discussed later).

- No eggs (or very few), unless you are pregnant (then, two per day).

- No artificial sweeteners at all except stevia or Lo Han (sorry, no honey either).

- Absolutely no soda pop, sports drinks, vitamin or mineral waters (commercial) – all are very acidic.

- No refined flours or breads with yeast (fungus).

- Eat no white potatoes or white rice.

- No peanuts, cashews, or corn (molds, fungus, aflatoxins).

- No fruits except fresh lemons, limes, or avocados (eat lots of these). Other fruits are sources of sugars that will feed your cancer.

- ***NO SUGAR OF ANY KIND – PERIOD!***

- No soy products, except if fermented or in Reliv™ Products.

Well, that's a start. I know, I know – what's left? Actually, lots.

WHAT YOU CAN AND MUST EAT

Fresh (organic, if possible) vegetables are alkaline and chock full of the nutrients that we all need to support and build up our immune systems. I would partake abundantly of spinach and broccoli, cauliflower and brussel sprouts (I know), cabbage and celery, red, yellow, and green peppers (call these fruits if you like), kale and asparagus, green beans and peas, egg plant and yellow squash, mustard greens and collards, okra and parsley, lettuce, carrots and watercress. Eat them raw and juice them. I would especially juice carrots and have several glasses per day with some of these other veggies to flavor. One caution. If you are on blood thinners, be careful of foods high in Vitamin K, using lower doses. You should consult your doctor on this, preferably a Naturopath.

Let me expound a little on one of nature's true superfoods and one listed as a "fruit" that I recommend highly – and in large quantities – for cancer sufferers. Commonly called an "alligator pear," the avocado, the harbinger of guacamole, is absolutely loaded with omega 3 and omega 6 fatty acids – of which most of us are deficient. Many people believe that, since avocados are high in fat, this nutritious food will, in turn, make them fat. Not so. This fruit has no cholesterol and its fats are, essentially, non-fattening.

The rich protein in avocados is predigested and gives up to the eater 18 essential amino acids needed for complete protein in the body. Full of magnesium, many other minerals, vitamins and enzymes, the avocado is truly one of the world's most "complete" foods. And, again, eat lots of them.

Organic, extra-virgin coconut oil, unlike most processed oils, is actually very good for you and loaded with healthy lauric acid. It tastes great, has a high smoke point (so you can cook with it), can be used as a butter substitute, and will store at room temperature for over a year without going bad. And please remember, almost all oils that you can buy from the grocery store are *already rancid* when you lift them from the shelf. Commercial perfumes have been added so they don't smell bad. I know, you can't believe this is true – but, sadly, it is. Don't buy or use any of these.

Several studies are telling us what we already know – olive oil prevents and fights cancer, especially breast cancer. I would use extra-virgin (the least possible processing and first pressed) in salads and as a supplement by the spoonful. Olive oil is also indicated as a preventative for heart disease, Parkinson's Disease, and Alzheimer's. Get plenty.

Here's a good one. The little known, often maligned, and seldom ingested vegetable, **watercress,** is having a great "coming-out" party. Jonathan Benson, a staff writer for *NaturalNews.com*, writes this about the secretive veggie:

> "New research out of the Cancer Research Centre at Southampton General Hospital's School of Medicine in the U.K. has found that watercress, a superfood vegetable, works to reduce levels of the key growth factor that causes tumor growth. According to researchers, regular consumption of watercress works the same as – if not better than – conventional anti-cancer drug treatments, except without all the harmful side effects."

I'm hoping you paid close attention to that last sentence. I am very sure that a similar paragraph could be written about most vegetables produced organically today. Vegetables are the true megafoods – and always have been. Make no mistake, if you want to heal from cancer, these largely ignored foods are the key.

Organic oatmeal is great with almond milk (organic unsweetened) and a little stevia. Eat beans for protein (not processed and sugared pork and beans), seeds (especially flax), and nuts (no peanuts or cashews). Have plenty of almonds, macadamia nuts and walnuts.

The primary nut/seed that I would consume would be apricot kernels. For those of you not familiar with these, they are about the size of an almond and come from inside the apricot pit. They are naturally dried and then packed and sold in many health food stores (in refrigerators) and on-line. You can get 2 pounds for about $25 or so (that's lots of seeds).

Apricot kernels are very high in Vitamin B-17, also known as amygdalin or Laetrile, and Vitamin B-15, also known as pangamic acid – both of which I believe are critical for cancer patients. Our government refuses to recognize these vitamins and has tried to outlaw them – so you know that they must be very effective at battling cancer. The Hunzakut people (Northern Pakistan) eat loads of apricot kernels and have never had a known case of cancer. I have eaten as many as 25 within a 10-minute period with no adverse reaction.

So that you know, many (including the American Cancer Society and our own government) will try to scare you into believing that these seeds will poison you and that there is no evidence that they have any effect on cancer. They are absolutely wrong on both counts and the evidence *against* them – and *for* this food – is incredibly overwhelming.

These seeds have a "locked" cyanide molecule (so do most other fruit seeds and Vitamin B-12) that is harmless to our normal cells but deadly to cancer cells. Our bodies have an enzyme (rhodanase) that neutralizes this molecule that the cancer cells lack (this is the short version – what you need to know). Many people claim that their cancers have been healed through apricot kernels alone. Go online and read Jason Vale's story at the following web address:

www.apricotsfromgod.info/mystory

Dr. Giuseppe Nacci, M.D., speaks volumes in a few short sentences about vitamin B17 (amygdalin/Laetrile):

"Give a seed of apple or other fruit to all the people you know, explaining to them that all fruit seeds contain vitamin B17; this vitamin cures cancer, a terrible disease deriving from a simple deficiency in vitamin B17…and other vitamins."

If you really want to know about the efficacy of Laetrile (amygdalin, apricot kernels), acquire the book *Laetrile Case Histories; The Richardson*

Cancer Clinic Experience, by Dr. John A. Richardson, M.D., and Patricia Irving Griffin, R.N., B.S. In this book you will discover 62 case histories that will prove to you – beyond any doubt whatsoever – that Laetrile (vitamin B17) works in the control and healing of cancer. Each single story is authenticated by a firm diagnosis and meticulous medical documentation.

What is very interesting is that this new updated version includes a follow-up 30 years after the patients were diagnosed with ***incurable cancer***. Proof is in the actual life-span of these people who previously had been told by their doctors that they had just a few months to live. This book also recounts the personal battle of Dr. Richardson who incurred the wrath of orthodox medicine when he and his patients elected to use vitamin therapy instead of surgery, drugs, and radiation as a treatment of choice.

This description of the book is from Ed Griffin's incredible website, www.realityzone.com, where you can find this astonishing work. Do go to this site regardless and view (and sign up for – it's free) one of the greatest and most informative newsletters of this generation – *The Reality Zone*.

Now, back to the apricot kernels. I would start with about 5 6 kernels per day and increase by one a day until getting to at least 18-20. The Vitamin B-15 (pangamic acid) in the seeds is known as "instant oxygen" and was heavily utilized by Russian athletes in the 60's-70's and beyond (remember how they excelled back then?). More oxygen, remember, is good for you and bad for cancer.

Another two foods that I would get plenty of – and that I believe are a "must" for cancer patients – are wheat grass and barley grass/leaves. Both of these contain all the essential amino acids and are rich in live enzymes, fiber, vitamins, minerals and chlorophyll. If you recall your plant biology, you will remember that chlorophyll is essentially the "blood" of plants. It is similar to the hemoglobin in our own blood but, instead of iron, it contains magnesium. And most of us are deficient in magnesium. The wheat grass can be a little difficult because you must juice it with a good juicing machine and you have to either raise it yourself or buy it at your local co-op, health food store, or through an Internet store. It is worth the trouble and, personally, I love the taste – a little sweet. You can also acquire it as a "frozen juice", in powder form, or tablets. Obviously, fresh-juiced is best – but these others will work, as well. Barley leaf or barley grass is best found as an organic supplement and I take it in pill form. I prefer Barley Power™ from Green Supreme – but do your research and find what works for you – and take lots.

In my opinion, a cancer patient must use these two foods in their diet. They not only are rich in nutrients and very alkaline, they help to detoxify the liver, neutralize pollutants, and improve oxygen supply. Don't go without them. I wouldn't.

Eat onions, garlic, ginger, turmeric, brown rice, millet and buckwheat. For a complete listing of what is allowed and to get the most in-depth look at what a "real" cancer diet should contain, go to the Cancer Tutor link at the following Internet address:

www.cancertutor.com/AltTreatments/Alt_Diet

I am a coffee drinker (small amount) like many Americans today. I do not, however, recommend coffee for cancer patients. It is normally much too acidic and puts unneeded stress on the adrenal glands. And I can hear the die-hard, lifetime coffee consumers screaming bloody murder right now. Bear with me for a moment.

For some time now I have made my morning coffee with 9.5 pH, ionized water and discovered that, after brewing, the pH is still between 7.0 and 7.5. Based upon this finding, and knowing that prying this caffeine fix away from an addicted, life-long imbiber is futile, I would concede a very small amount – made as above – for those who would succumb to their recently ended addiction prior to their cancer. Given that fact, and having just seen the earth move above my great-grandmother's grave, I offer now a better suggestion.

At the Cancer Control Society's 38th Annual Convention over Labor Day in Universal City, California (this is a premier event – you should go), I visited a booth that was marketing (and giving samples of) a new coffee called Ganoderma.

Ganoderma Lucidum is the scientific name for a species of red mushrooms (Red Reishi) that have grown wild for thousands of years in Asia. This mushroom is said to have more than 200 active elements known to improve health – and I believe it. A super antioxidant, Ganoderma works mightily to strengthen the immune system (cancer patients need this) and helps with stress, toxins, infections, and improves circulation and respiration. It is currently being studied and researched as a *treatment* for cancer and other diseases.

The coffee itself is made from premium quality coffee beans, combined with the Ganoderma Lucidum, and produces a very rich blend and aroma that – I can personally say – is excellent and almost identical to my regular morning cup. The final product is alkaline, not acid, and is actually very good for you. While many companies are advertising similar products, my brand comes from Gano Excel and is their Ganocafe Classic. Get additional info at www.GanoExcel.us. Choose what you like and go for it.

For a cookbook for cancer patients visit this site:

www.cancerfreefoods.com

One of the greatest "recipe" books I have seen is entitled *Change Your Food...Change Your Life – 101 Recipes for an Alkaline Lifestyle* and is by my new friends, Sue and Barry Wilcox, from Montana. Cancer patients often complain that the new "cancer diet" leaves them nothing enjoyable to eat.

Absolutely not so – and within the 76 pages of this work Sue and Barry prove me right.

From salads and dressings to main dishes, breads, snacks and desserts, this couple has mastered the nearly impossible task of combining excellent nutrition with superb taste. Please note – and they do – that cancer patients should go easy on cooked recipes and major in raw foods. Follow their 80/20 rule: "Eighty percent of every meal should be fresh, raw or lightly steamed. Twenty percent of every meal can be cooked or slightly acidic."

And here is a bit of wisdom from Sue and Barry regarding plant-based foods and their nutrients that refutes (factually and righteously so) the myth that one must get their protein from animal products:

"What about protein and calcium? Many people wonder where we obtain these important nutrients if we limit our animal protein products. In short, all green leafy vegetables and grasses provide a substantial amount of calcium as well as iron, magnesium, vitamin C, and many of the B vitamins. Plant-based foods have a much greater nutrient composition than animal-based foods. The main protein foods in a vegan diet are: (1) pulses – the edible seed of peas, beans and lentils; (2) nuts; (3) seeds; and (4) grains – all of which are relatively energy dense. Pulses average 27 percent of calories from protein. Nuts and seeds average 13 percent of calories from protein, grains average 12 percent. Plant foods can supply the recommended amount of protein if you are making good choices."

We can understand the folly of believing only good protein comes from animals (meat, milk, etc.) when we look out into a field flowing with green grass and see a muscular, half-ton bull who – to my knowledge – has never eaten a steak or dined on a pork chop. Life's funny that way. It appears that this "vegan" animal has done just fine on his "greens."

Sue and Barry Wilcox are Nutritional Coaches and Educators and have been conducting nutritional cooking clinics since 2003. Barry is certified in Nutritional Microscopy by the Intermountain Institute of Natural Health. They know their stuff and have invested over three decades in bringing this recipe guide to the general public. You can find them and their recipe book at www.healthywaystocook.com.

Please note to use the recipes that are in line with the "cancer diet" protocol in this chapter – most of them will be. Be innovative and make it work for you. I have no financial interest in either of the above sites and receive no remuneration for these cook book and recipe book recommendations. Actually, the same goes for any endorsements or recommendations in this book.

SALT AND PEPPER

We are not going to spend a lot of time on black pepper. Just know that it is very acidic and should be avoided by cancer patients.

Salt is, however, a very different story. We have been advised by our doctors and T.V. sets to avoid it or significantly reduce our intake at all costs. Salt is purported to be directly related to high blood pressure, heart disease, and almost all other sickness known to man. Now, here are the facts:

Table salt (sodium chloride), stripped of all its minerals, blanched, bleached – and who knows what else – is indeed not good for you and may certainly cause and contribute to the medical conditions mentioned above. As a result, many are turning to "sea salt" and declaring that it is good. Be advised that herein, the deception begins. You see, all salt is "sea salt" as it originally came from the sea. The problem arises when man gets hold of it and reduces it to sodium chloride and, perhaps, some synthetic iodine.

I would not eat any salt that was white. Instead, I would look for a "full spectrum salt" – one that is original and unadulterated – containing all the basic 84 additional minerals that it was born with. Full spectrum salt is, essentially, a health food. Your body actually "requires" it. These salts contain minerals in the same concentration as your blood does. They increase energy by improving cellular communication, help eliminate cellular toxins and improve nutrient absorption.

Friends, full-spectrum salt is truly organic – dug from the ancient sea caves and virtually not processed, allowing it to keep its health and healing attributes intact. I use Himalayan Salt and it is a reddish brown color. Make sure your salt has color – indicating that it has not been stripped or processed and the minerals are still there.

THE BUDWIG PROTOCOL

The key ingredient of an oxygen and alkaline-rich cancer diet is – and has been for some time – the now, world-famous, "Budwig protocol." It is so-named for the woman who researched and discovered the miracle of combining the omega 3 fats of flax oil with the sulfurated protein of organic, low-fat cottage cheese. This one formula has probably helped (and healed) more suffering cancer patients than any other food, supplement, or anti-cancer protocol – or any combinations thereof.

Although simple in its design and ingredients, the complexity of how it works is beyond the scope of this book. Suffice it to say that the fats and proteins, when mixed thoroughly, produce a mechanism to "unlock" or open up the cancer cells and force in oxygen. Remember, cancer hates oxygen and cannot survive in its presence. Listen: it works, and there are literally thousands of testimonies to prove it.

The recipe calls for an approximate 2 to 1 ratio of the basic two ingredients – two heaping tablespoons of cottage cheese for every tablespoon of organic flax oil (preferably not high lignin). I recommend organic, low-fat cottage cheese from your local health food store and Barlean's™ brand flax oil (I believe it to be the freshest and best – but choose what you like). Always refrigerate both, however, whatever you choose.

Mix the cottage cheese and flax oil (also called linseed oil) with a spoon then with an immersion blender (hand held). Now, this next step is really important. In order to be effective, these two must be blended well enough to virtually become one substance – almost like whipped cream. Thirty seconds to a minute should do it. Next, grind up some fresh brown flax seeds (with a small coffee grinder) and mix them in. Grind only what you will use for that portion because they will go rancid after grinding if left too long. Refrigerate the remainder of the "whole" flax seeds. You can add fresh lemon or lime juice, Vietnamese cinnamon, or some stevia to flavor, and ground almonds, walnuts or macadamia nuts. Let the completed mixture sit for five to ten minutes prior to consumption, to allow the "chemical reaction" to take place. I have eaten it plain (with no additives) and it doesn't taste bad at all. If you absolutely cannot handle the flavor, you can add a couple of blueberries, raspberries, strawberries, etc., if you must. Go easy on these. Eat a half-cup to a cup (at least) of the mixture twice a day.

I have been told that cottage cheese ceases being a dairy product once it is mixed with the flax oil. I cannot prove that – but it makes no difference. I believe this protocol to be a "must" for a cancer patient. I would make this a primary and daily regimen of my anti-cancer diet.

To see a short video of how to prepare this "meal", go to the link below and scroll down to "Dr. Johanna Budwig's Healing Diet and Protocol" and click on the video:

www.americanaci.org/articlepage.aspx?categoryID=46

As of this writing, there has been published a "Budwig Diet Revision" paper that calls for different ingredients based upon, essentially, the same science. This "revision" calls for cold-processed whey instead of cottage cheese, and wild salmon oil in lieu of flax oil. I have reviewed this new protocol (and have looked at other opinions) and the data behind it appears to be very controversial, at a minimum. I believe that whey and wild salmon oil can be a good part of a balanced diet. At this time, however, without the reams of empirical evidence that the Budwig Diet boasts, I would not "switch" to the revision and would not consider adding it to my anti-cancer routine. Investigate for yourself.

CONCLUSION

What you eat (and don't eat) during the length of your cancer "experience" will make a significant difference to the eventual outcome. Many people have been known to heal their cancer through diet alone. I have personally talked to a 70-year-old woman who was diagnosed with pancreatic cancer at about age 40. She followed a "diet only" treatment plan and resolved her "doctor diagnosed death sentence" on her own – in relatively short order. She was alive and well when I spoke with her a couple of years ago, some 30 years after that event.

Please, don't tell me that diet is not that important, and don't listen to those who do. We know that many doctors don't believe that it plays any part in this disease but – on this count – they are simply wrong. With cancer, the significance of diet cannot be understated. It can literally make you or break you. The correct cancer diet will alkalinize and oxygenate your body, which can essentially stop the growth of (and kill – or revert) cancer cells. This protocol will also "feed" the good cells that are critical to your recovery.

While there are no guarantees, most people who flee conventional treatments and embrace a proper nutrient-dense, alkaline and oxygen rich diet – get well. If I had cancer, I would definitely get on the right diet protocol. And I have no doubt that it would be the key to strengthening my immune system and healing me.

Oh, one last thing. NO CHOCOLATE. Sorry.

CHAPTER FIVE

"STEP TWO OF THE CANCER DIET: SUPPLEMENTS"

"If you have had breast cancer, if you are at high risk for breast cancer, if you are afraid of getting breast cancer, or if you are just smart, you will take cod liver oil for the rest of your life."

Dr. Bruce West – *Health Alert*

WHILE the right food and water are the baseline for stopping your cancer in its tracks, it will be a combination of unique supplemental, nutritional products that turn it around.

Mentioning "supplements" to someone can conjure up all kinds of visions. At one time or another, we have all been introduced to lotions, potions and elixirs with attached claims that usually don't materialize. Hence, a multitude have jumped from one product or one company to another in search of the "Holy Grail" of health and healing, while many others have just given up.

The truly encouraging part of this is the reality that, as many abandon the quest, others are finding that the "supplement world" is now producing some real game changing – and life changing – products. What is particularly interesting to those of us that forward "alternatives" – and particularly dismaying to conventional researchers and allopathic medicine – is the fact that these supplements are coming from natural sources, are non-toxic, have virtually no "side effects", build the immune system, and are actually good for you.

You see, pharmaceutical companies make their billions by taking natural elements and compounds, i.e., taxol from the Pacific Yew tree to make the drug Paclitaxel (or Abraxane) (yuk!), synthesize them into unnatural compounds that may suppress some symptoms but have no healing or normalizing capacity (and multitudes of terrible side effects), test them marginally, declare them good, then sell the paperwork to the FDA for approval. The process becomes complete when you take the pill that, ultimately, will produce other maladies within your body which require more pills – and on it goes.

Imagine the conundrum when a major drug company discovered graviola in the Brazilian Rain Forest. Remember the movie "Medicine Man" with Sean Connery and you will get the connection. Well, shortening the story, this company took the leaves, branches, bark, roots, and flowers from this tree (graviola) and used the extracts from them "in vitro" (petri dishes and test tubes) to determine their effect on cancer cells. Guess what? The extracts killed all the cancer they came into contact with. So, naturally, the next step for a good drug company would be to **not** offer the inexpensive extract to people to cure their cancer. For Heaven's sakes, there's no money in that! No, the stuff had to be synthesized into a drug that could be patented and sold for billions.

The problem was that "Mother Nature" was too smart for the drug researchers. You see, God already had the patent on this stuff. They were simply not able to make it into a drug that would do what the raw extract would. So, once again, like a responsible pharmaceutical company should, they buried the research so nobody could have it – about eight years after they started. And just how many other "graviolas" do you think are out there?

To finish the account of this now well-publicized cover-up, eventually an employee who had worked on the project (as this story is told) left the company and spilled the beans. Supplement companies jumped on it, headed to the rainforest, harvested, tested and produced an extract that is a "natural chemotherapy" – a harmless agent that is said to be 10,000 times more effective than toxic chemotherapeutic drugs – but, alas, with no side effects. You can buy graviola on the open market now, but the American Cancer Society and all other governmental agencies will tell you that it doesn't do anything and is ineffective. This, my friends, is the real problem with supplements today. Many work wonders but are not allowed to see the light of day by the "powers that be."

Go to the ACS website and check in under "Complimentary and Alternative Therapies – Pharmacological and Biological Treatment." What you will find is a host of "alternative" treatments, each with its corresponding explanation and evaluation. Almost all of the data will say something to the effect that, "available scientific evidence does not suggest that 'XXX' is effective in treating cancer in humans." Yeah, right. And chemotherapy is. There is no scientific evidence because all "allopathic truth" (under their own law of scientific evidence) must be produced by clinical trials that cost hundreds of millions of dollars. And the FDA, et al., knows that no one is going to pay that kind of money to clinically test a natural product that cannot be patented. End of story.

To be fair, many supplements sold today are not worth the bottles that they are sold in. You really must be careful and undertake your own due diligence here. Study up. Please, don't settle for supermarket-bought synthetic vitamins, "super juices" of unknown origin, or unproven technology of any kind. Supplements for a cancer patient are critical – why would you skimp or settle? Don't do it.

Frankly, I recommend very few supplements. I've just told you why. What I will present to you next are the exact products (supplements) that I would use if I had cancer. These are not "type of cancer" specific (with the exception of some protomorphogens). I've said it before, and I'll say it again – and some will want to argue with me – but they won't win. ***Cancer is cancer.*** There are different classes and kinds, names and definitions, and many and various sites where it is found. For the most part, however, with very few exceptions or additions, it is all treated and healed the same way – by giving the body what it needs to normalize itself.

Good supplements play a critical part in this cellular equalization. We can disagree about how you acquired your disease or how your doctor describes it, but there should be no arguing that you must do ***whatever*** is logical, effective and (naturally) necessary to rid yourself of it. With all cancer, the immune system is weakened and it must be restored if you are to have a chance, regardless of whether you have melanoma, liver cancer or ductal carcinoma in-situ. So, it doesn't matter what "type" or what "name" you put on it. What matters is that you make the right decisions and engage in the appropriate procedures that will enable your body to kill it. Enough said.

There are literally thousands of nutritional and topical supplements in the marketplace today that are available for purchase through several different mediums. No matter how you acquire them, you must make sure that you are getting those that have real empirical proof behind them – not "borrowed" or "adopted" science. What this means, simply, is that the data, testing, and evidence supporting the product is for that individual entity itself – not for a generalized or similar category. For example, synthetic Vitamin E is not – nor should it be compared with – natural, mixed tocopherols. Similarly, ascorbic acid is not the whole Vitamin C complex. Fractionated vitamins do not include all of the supporting elements and nutrients found in organic whole foods. And so on and so forth. Please, do not waste your hard-earned dollars on any single item that will not be efficacious for your health or healing – especially if you have the challenge of cancer.

PHYTONUTRIENTS/PROTOMORPHOGENS

Speaking of vitamins, I would try to get the majority of these and the necessary minerals and enzymes through the whole foods that I would now be eating on the proper cancer diet. Then, I would supplement with organic phytonutrients (from plants) that provide the entire realm of vitamins, minerals, enzymes and activators, and organ/tissue-specific protomorphogens (tissue extracts) that contain "the tiniest specks of life" made specifically by your body for each kind of tissue. Most of us are pretty familiar with phytonutrients, but have very little or no understanding of PMGs (protomorphogens). Let's go to "PMG 101" to find out exactly what they are and what they do within the human body – especially for cancer patients.

According to Dr. Bruce West, here is what you need to know about PMGs:

"Verified by scientists, including Bechamp, Rife, Beadle, Northrup, Robertson, Turck, and others, the theory of PMGs sheds light on how the body controls its own cell growth and heals itself. When viewed under a special microscope like that used by Royal Rife or Gaston Naessens, human blood teems with super-active life in the form of the smallest particles imaginable – PMGs. The same blood under any other microscope, even the electron microscope, appears almost dead with only the red corpuscles, platelets, white cells, etc., being viewed.

"When injury or disease to a tissue, gland, or organ occurs, the body's production of PMGs changes. These specks of life kick into high gear and control the healing process. They are involved in the way the body produces antibodies and they maintain the health of the tissue. According to the theory, in cancer the PMG blueprint is altered and cell reproduction goes on uncontrolled. Without regaining some control, the result is ever-expanding cancer and tumors.

"Lee (Dr. Royal Lee) knew that humans could 'borrow' certain body materials from animals. Examples include thyroid hormone from pigs and female hormone from horses. He developed patented equipment (he held more than 75 patents) to actually extract the PMG material from animal glands, tissues, and organs. He did this for 23 tissues, producing PMG supplements that were processed without heat, maintaining their specific blueprint integrity and function.

"By taking PMGs of the diseased tissue by mouth, it was soon discovered they had a healing and controlling influence for the patient suffering from the disease. This was proven with lab tests, x-rays, and functional analyses. And for the patient with cancer, PMG therapy is absolutely essential. In fact, without adequate PMGs (either from within the body or from supplements), chances of surviving cancer are nil." *Health Alert*, Special Report #3-5, Dr. Bruce West.

Folks, listen to this doctor. I have, I did, and I do. Doctor Bruce West has probably helped heal more heart patients than any doctor – dead or alive. He knows what he is talking about with regard to disease and supports and recommends these phytonutrients and protomorphogens to patients suffering from every ailment known to man – including cancer. The supplements that he recommends (and that I take) are, largely, from the company known as Standard Process™. Their lineup of over 160 whole food products is mostly grown organically on their own farm in Palmyra, Wisconsin – and has been since 1929. Some raw organic product is bought outside. These supplements are sold exclusively through "health care professionals", and many of those appear to be "on-line" (find them there). I have procured mine through Dr. West's company, Health Alert, and have been very satisfied with their service. Dr. West has no stake in

Standard Process™; he desires only to offer the best products that make a real change in patient's lives. I also have no financial interest in recommending these supplements or Dr. West.

If I had cancer (even if I didn't), I would be on these phytonutrient and protomorphogen products immediately. I would also subscribe (and I do) to Dr. West's Newsletter, *Health Alert*, as it is chock-full of what I like to call "the real truth about disease and healing." I feel it's a bargain at 10 times the price and goes for only $39 per year. Reach his office at 831-372-2103 or 888-525-5955 and website at www.healthalert.com. Again, I have no financial or other interest here (save getting you what you need to heal).

ALOE ARBORESCENS

Most people have heard of aloe and some still keep a potted aloe vera plant for the purpose of slathering its healing gel on a burn or abrasion, but very few know of aloe arborescens – even though the first record of its pharmacological use was found on a sumeric tablet dating back to 2100 B.C. Aren't we paying attention (sorry)? With this derivative of aloe, there is a long history of study, research and use – but you can review that at another time. What you need to know right now is that this variety of aloe is said to have a 300% *stronger curative potential* than aloe vera.

Father Romano Zago, a Brazilian Catholic Friar, is the one generally credited with bringing the knowledge about aloe arborescens to the world. His is another interesting story about unselfish service and dutiful research, and he has recently forwarded this life changing preparation and written about how to make and administer the healing concoction.

His original formula consists of juice from organically grown and timely harvested (five-year-old) aloe arborescens leaves, unheated, pesticide-free raw honey, and 1% certified organic alcohol for effective absorption. Dosage calls for 2-3 tablespoons per day consumed 20-30 minutes before a meal on an empty stomach. It can be taken for ten days on and ten days off – or steadily until the condition is resolved (cancer). You can find the story of this incredible product and the original recipe (in Father Zago's own words) at www.aloearborescens.org/Summary.pdf or by purchasing his book, *Cancer Can Be Cured*, at Amazon.com. Also, you can find excellent information about this extract and homeopathic solution at the following website page:

http://cancertutor.com/Cancer03/AloeArborescens

Aloe arborescens is an anti-inflammatory, pain inhibitor, anti-fungal, anti-microbial, immune system builder – and the rest of the list of its health-inducing properties is many pages long. It contains 4 times as many enzymes as aloe vera, 20 amino acids, and is a virtual cornucopia of essential minerals and vitamins.

If I had cancer (or not), I would immediately acquire and begin ingesting this supplement. Make it yourself or find a good source. Deca Aloe Arborescens U.S., markets the original formula that is endorsed by Father Zago. Actually, the Deca Arborescens Galenia® mixture is the only brand that is authorized to carry Father Zago's signature and picture on the label to vouch for the authenticity of the exacting recipe. You can procure their product, Galenia® Aloe Arborescens, through their website at the following address:

www.aloedeca.com

As is the case in all the product recommendations in this book, I receive no remuneration and have no financial relationships with the vendors.

TRANSFER FACTORS

Transfer "what?" Actually, it is probably something that we should all know about – but we don't. When a baby is born, its first food is generally its mother's milk. Transfer factors are essentially immune system molecules that are transferred from mother to child in the "colostrum" or "first milk" of this process that effectively establishes the immune system of the newborn.

In its purest sense, transfer factor is a natural substance that teaches the immune system to identify and kill infectious agents within the body. These "factors" are also present in the colostrum of cows and goats. This "first milk after birth" is collected, transfer factor molecules are obtained, dried and, subsequently, encapsulated in an "all natural" form for human consumption.

Over 3,000 papers have been published on transfer factors and more than 50 years of research has been done. There are virtually thousands of testimonies to its efficacy and immune building proclivity. A recent "blinded cytoxicity" study showed that transfer factors increased Natural-Killer Cell effectivity by 248% (Independent NK Cell Study Report, Calvin W. McCausland, Ph.D., Emma Oganova, M.D., Ph.D.). Another study involving transfer factor testing revealed inducement of immune-based lysis (breaking down or destruction of cells) of K562 cells (erythro leukemia cell line) at unprecedented levels (Institute of Longevity Medicine, California, 11.05.99).

A study on 20 Stage IV (late stage) cancer patients (12 males, 8 females) with physician prognosis of approximately 3.7 months to live showed a remarkable result. Of these 20 patients who were supposed to die in less than 4 months, 16 were alive, in remission, and prospering a year later. They were given transfer factors, digestive enzymes and beta glucans – immune system boosters (study by D. See, S. Mason, R. Roshan, Center for Advanced Medicine, Encinitas, CA, 2002).

As you recall, a strong immune system is really the only way to beat cancer. It has the ability, it has the strength, it can do the job – but only if it is "fed" the proper foods, water and supplemental nutrients that will allow it to do so. It is beyond any doubt that transfer factors establish and boost the immune system and, if I had cancer, I wouldn't be without them.

The Camelot Cancer Care Center in Tulsa, Oklahoma (which I highly recommend for cancer patients – contact Maureen Long), is doing incredible work involving goat colostrum at its new facility in Cancun, Mexico. Theirs is a cutting-edge transfer factor technique and treatment that is protected under the Mexican Constitution via the Mayan/Aztec healing heritage laws because it is blood/colostrum (milk) based – which is different from transfer factors that are available in the United States. In a recent visit with Maureen, I learned all about this fascinating new technology. It is, however, beyond the scope of this book.

Bottom line: I would definitely involve transfer factors in my "alternative" treatment for cancer. Contact the parent company, 4Life, at www.4life.com. They will take care of you regarding these supplements.

COLLOIDAL SILVER

I'm always surprised to find out that most people still do not know the story of colloidal silver or "silver water" and its healing properties.

Silver has been around forever and our ancestors knew of its wondrous capabilities. Pioneers in covered wagons placed silver dollars (coins really made of silver) in their milk and water to retard bacterial growth. It was used in the late 1800's to prevent eye disease and in the early 1900's in wound dressings and for burns. The discovery of antibiotics drove silver from the marketplace despite the fact that silver was – and is – much more effective than these drugs, and pathogens cannot build an immunity to it. Silver is currently being used in burn centers (to some degree) and silver fibers are being woven into outdoor and sports clothing to inhibit odor-causing bacterial growth. It is also utilized in washing machines for the same reason.

For example, Samsung recently introduced a clothes washing machine that kills 99% of bacteria in cold water by using silver ions. Addidas and Polartec have licensed a silver-coated nylon fabric known as X-Static™ that incorporates germ-killing silver into athletic and outdoor clothing. Curad and Johnson and Johnson offer bandages with ionic silver impregnated into the gauze. AcryMed, a nanotechnology company, recently announced FDA approval of its SilvaGard™, a silver nanotech coating to protect medical devices from bacteria. Nexxion makes ionic silver coatings for catheters, I.V. needles, and other medical devices. "To date, no pathogens have been able to survive contact with silver." Silver data is from the April 17, 2006 edition of *Chemical and Engineering News*, and the quote from Bethany Halford and her article entitled, "A Silver Bullet for Infections," from the same source.

Silver is proven – but not yet approved by the FDA for internal medical applications. Hence, no claims can be made for it. Colloidal and ionic silver are basically solutions of microscopic silver particles suspended in pure (distilled) water. These substances kill microbes and bacteria, and strengthen the immune system. There are many, many testimonies about their healing properties and anti-cancer abilities. Many people drink from an ounce to a quart a day. And no, properly made and used elemental silver water and ionic silver solutions do not turn your skin blue (argyria).

If I had cancer I would be drinking this stuff. Come to think of it – I drink it anyway and I'm well and don't look like a "smurf". You can buy this in 8 ounce to quart bottles or make it yourself by acquiring a silver generator. The generators are not that expensive and will save you lots of money in the long run. You can buy the bottled product on line or through your local health food store. Just get a good brand. Find a good ionic or colloidal silver product that is 10 20 parts per million of silver and make sure that it is crystal clear (pure) with no yellow or blue coloring. If you believe that you want to try a generator, go to the following website: www.silvermedicine.org/colloidal-silver-generators.html - and get the full scoop. You probably can't drink too much of this – but I would start slowly, maybe an ounce or two a few times a day, and then build from there as you are comfortable with it.

CELLECT™

My initial feeling about recommending Cellect™ as an anti-cancer supplement is that I should advise you to just go and get it – no matter what it takes or what it costs – it's that important. Many cancer coaches that I know make it an integral part of the cancer diet and incorporate it with the Budwig protocol. Cellect™ is, in essence, a concoction that combines a powdered mix of vitamins, minerals, shark cartilage, milk thistle, gelatin and other ingredients with cod liver oil capsules to produce a dietary supplement that is a significant immune system booster that many say has helped to cure their cancer. This product balances your body chemically and nutritionally and there are some that believe it just flat kills cancer cells.

Cellect™ was invented by Fred Eichorn, President of the National Cancer Research Foundation. Fred watched his sister die of cancer while undergoing traditional treatments – then cured his own pancreatic cancer using no conventional therapies. Fred's belief is that "the cause (of cancer) is the result of the nutritional deficiency altering the environmental source, which, upon re-establishing the correct nutritional levels in the body, the environment would be corrected for normal body functions and no longer be provisional to the cancer's survival, hence, the cancer will soon die as a result." Got that? Read "nutritional deficiency", "re-establishing", "cancer will soon die". It makes good sense.

I think everyone really knew that Fred was onto something when we heard that he was visited by the FDA. This is what happens when you become a threat to the conventional cancer industry – the lucrative business of surgery, drugs, chemo and radiation therapies.

Cellect™ is rather expensive at about $80 per can (30 servings). And you really need a lot of it to make a difference. It is very cheap, however, compared to an average day in the hospital for a cancer patient – now over $6,000. And, no, don't be fooled into thinking that insurance pays for it all (traditional cancer treatment) – even if you have insurance. The largest cause of bankruptcies in the United States today is the result of uninsured or "non-covered" medical costs. And most of those are because of cancer bills that have gone unpaid because insurance "didn't cover it all." Homes are lost, vehicles repossessed, personal property sold at pennies on the dollar. Still, many cancer sufferers find themselves not able to pay the ever-rising cancer costs of conventional medicine. It shouldn't be so. No, compared to this, Cellect™ and almost all other "alternative" cancer treatments, supplements, and protocols are very inexpensive. And they work.

Take this product immediately before a meal and the cod liver oil capsules during the meal (thanks, Webster). Build up to 4 scoops a day – if you can. No, it doesn't taste that great. Mix it with a freshly juiced vegetable "cocktail", guzzle it down, and be happy. If you have any constipation with this, increase the amount of cod liver oil and drink more fresh juices. Separate the ingestion of this with the Budwig Protocol by two hours.

You can purchase Cellect™ through their website located at www. cellect.org. You can find the protocol on how to take this at www.cancer-tutor.com/Cancer02/cellect_Budwig.html. Also, enter "National Cancer Research Foundation" into your search engine to get the entire Cellect™ story. I would.

MAGNESIUM CHLORIDE

"If we looked it would probably be very difficult to find a cancer patient with anywhere near normal levels of cellular magnesium – meaning cancer probably does not exist in a physical cellular environment full of magnesium." (From the Magnesium For Life website). Wow! What an outrageous statement. Nonetheless, I believe it to be true.

The preceding site follows up with this: "Magnesium chloride is the first and most important item in any person's cancer treatment strategy. Put in the clearest terms possible, our suggestion from the first day on the *Survival Medicine Cancer Protocol* is to almost drown oneself in transdermally (through the skin – topically) applied magnesium chloride. It should be the first – not the last – thing we think of when it comes to cancer. It takes about three to four months to drive up cellular magnesium levels to where they should be when treated intensely transdermally, but within days patients will commonly experience its life saving medical/ healing effects. For many people whose bodies are starving for magnesium the experience is not too much different than for a person coming out of a desert desperate for water. It is that basic to life, that important, that necessary." Gee, they just got bolder! And, once again, I agree with them.

When you understand that magnesium is a magnificent cellular detoxifier and tissue purifier, that it is necessary for many enzyme reactions and less toxic than table salt – you see clearly why many call it the "miracle mineral."

In 1915, French surgeon Pierre Delbet discovered that white blood cells destroyed up to three times more microbes after the intake of magnesium chloride. Early stage polio and diphtheria have been "cured" by magnesium chloride. The research and evidence behind this substance are truly incredible (see the following site for the studies):

www.magnesiumforlife.com/medical-application/ magnesium-and-cancer

Shirley Lipschutz-Robinson of Shirley's Wellness Café, says that "nothing short of a miracle is to be expected in ones health status if one is ill when one increases the cellular levels of magnesium." And Shirley knows what she is talking about. Read about Shirley's Wellness Journey by entering "Shirley's Wellness Café" into your search engine.

And the coup de grace for those suffering from the pain of cancer – again from the Magnesium For Life website: "Magnesium chloride, when applied directly to the skin, is transdermally absorbed and has an almost immediate effect on chronic and acute pain." Tell me, how important is that?

The evidence is in, folks. The case for magnesium chloride has been presented over the last 150 years. It has been accused of helping those suffering from cancer by significantly improving their immune function, reducing their pain, and increasing their cellular detoxification. The Verdict? Guilty, as charged. Now go get you some.

I recommend ultra-pure magnesium chloride that is drawn from the Ancient Zechstein Seabed in Northern Europe. It is naturally fortified with other trace minerals and available from Ancient Minerals, the number one brand for topical magnesium therapy in the world. Find them and the magnesium chloride oil at www.ancient-minerals.com. This product comes in 8 ounce ($29) and 64 ounce ($119) sizes. For what it is and what it does – this price is like stealing it. If I had cancer (or any other challenging medical problem), I would order it right now before I finished this book. Do finish this book, however.

For an in-depth study of magnesium chloride, visit the Magnesium For Life website at www.magnesiumforlife.com.

GLUTATHIONE

Glutathione is called the "master anti-oxidant" and is a tri-peptide, or a combination of three amino acids – cysteine, glycine, and glutamic acid. It must be generated inside the cells from its "precursors" before it can do its work effectively. In other words, the body makes it itself and you cannot just buy and consume a glutathione supplement. Any such-labeled product would, instead, be one of the amino acid precursors – most likely cysteine in whey protein.

Proof of its anti-oxidant and anti-cancer capability comes from a study at Montreal General Hospital and McGill University in Montreal that suggests "whey protein may be exerting its effect on carcinogens by enhancing glutathione concentration," (Gold, Batist, Bounous, *Immuno-enhancing Property of Diet and Whey Protein*, 1989).

According to the "Nutrition Advisor" website, "Glutathione is a substance, the levels of which in our cells are predictive of how long we will live. There are very few other factors which are as predictive of our life expectancy as is our level of cellular glutathione. Glutathione has been called the 'master antioxidant' and regulates the actions of lesser antioxidants such as vitamin C and vitamin E within the body. It is the regulator and regenerator of immune cells and the most valuable detoxifying agent in the human body." View 23 published clinical studies on glutathione at this site: www.nutritionadvisor.com/glutathione.html.

It is the immune system that ultimately heals a cancerous body. And glutathione plays a (or "the") major role in the "cranking up" and maintenance of this system. We literally can't be without it and, unfortunately, most of us don't have – or make – nearly enough. Production of this cancer fighting antioxidant diminishes as we age and is also determined by what we eat and how we live our lives.

Dr. Earl Mindell (*The Vitamin Bible*) states candidly that "we literally cannot survive without this antioxidant." Cancer patients ***absolutely*** cannot. Time to go get it. I would – if I had cancer.

There are a few sources of glutathione precursors and you are free to investigate and choose which supplement works best for you. I recommend three – the first two are proven precursors and the third is a different technology that has verified its effectiveness through a clinical trial – and I forward it with a caveat. Immunocal ™ is a precursor with a natural source of cystein. You can purchase it at www.immunotec.com. It is a little costly (but worth it) at $90 for a container of 30 each, 10-gram pouches – about a month's supply. You can get a 20% discount if you sign up for an "auto ship" so it comes to you directly each month. Immunocal™ has some very impressive credentials and persuasive testimonies standing behind it.

MaxGXL, is a composition patented natural supplement that has been clinically tested and blood-test verified to raise the body's intracellular glutathione level 300% within 60 days. This product was invented by Dr. Robert Keller, M.D., and has great clinical documentation to support it. MaxGXL is available through the company website at www.maxgxl.com or through individual distributors. Retail price is about $85 for a month's supply – wholesale is about $65.

The new glutathione technology is from LifeWave, LLC. It is a gluta-thione "patch" that had a "coming out" in Suzanne Somers' new book, *Knockout*. The patch is affixed to various acupuncture points on the body and worn each day for up to twelve hours. The double-blind, placebo-controlled study showed an increase of over 300% in blood glutathione levels in 24 hours.

The LifeWave website gives the following description: "The materials in the patches consist of a patent-pending blend of water, oxygen, amino acids and organics applied to a polyester fabric and sealed with a polymer shell. The active materials are applied to a substrate so as to form a nano-scale organic antenna. When properly assembled, we believe that these LifeWave antennas are capable of passively communicating with the user to instruct or initiate various metabolic responses in the user."

There appears to be many testimonies from wearers that attest to the effectiveness of these patches. And the clinical study bears proof (at least in this case). The patches can't hurt you and carry a 30-day money back guarantee – so you can't lose. The "caveat" on this source is only because it is a relatively new technology and, although proven, I would like to see more empirical evidence and user support. It's definitely worth a go and I would try "the patch" if I had cancer.

Go to www.lifewave.com to order. A box of 30 (one month supply) goes for $79.90. Also, take into consideration that the cancer diet provides glutathione precursors abundantly in asparagus, broccoli, avocado, spinach, garlic, and turmeric. Eat these first – in quantity – then go for the precursor supplements.

POLY-MVA

Although it is not technically a "newcomer" to the anti-cancer scene, Poly-MVA is rapidly becoming one of the favorites of alternative treatment because of its huge success in late stage cancer.

Most of you have probably never heard of it – so let me tell you what it is first. Poly-MVA is a special combination of the element palladium and alpha lipoic acid (poly) along with molybdenum, rhodium, and ruthenium (minerals and elements), vitamins B1, B2, and B12 (vitamins), and formyl-methionine and N-acetylcysteine (amino acids); hence, the name Poly-MVA. Don't be fooled by its chemical makeup – these are all natural substances.

Most importantly, what this supplement brings to the table for cancer patients is powerful and effective. Poly-MVA enhances the function of the mitochondria – the "powerhouse" and main source of energy within the cells. It protects cells from damage and also increases their activity and function. Poly-MVA supports the liver (the main detoxification organ), helps remove heavy metals, is a super antioxidant, oxygenates the cells, and enhances the function of the white blood cells. And when you think of it, all of these are exactly what cancer patients require.

Over the past decade, the testimonials regarding this product and its ability to help the body heal itself – especially with cancer patients – are legion. In Chapter Ten you will read the healing story of Jessica Biscardi, a metastatic breast cancer survivor and star of the T.V. show, "The Incurables," who used a cancer diet and Poly-MVA to bring herself back from the brink of death.

Dr. James Forsythe, whom I met at the Cancer Control Society Convention in 2010, is the founder and director of the Century Wellness Clinic in Reno, Nevada, and a staunch supporter of Poly-MVA. Dr. Forsythe says that this product basically "turns up the voltage in cancer cells causing them to self-electrocute themselves" (paraphrase of actual quote).

If I had cancer, this is one product that I would absolutely fit into my anti-cancer regimen, particularly if I had late stage cancer. Poly-MVA is rather expensive at about $150 per 8-ounce bottle. Conversely, it's rather cheap for what it just might do for a cancer sufferer. Eight ounces could last up to three months – but it is more likely to be a one or two week supply when battling this severe disease. It's well worth it, however, and it is definitely what I would do.

MORINGA

There is a reason that they call Moringa the "Miracle Tree." It might be because all parts of the plant are edible. It might be that it has the ability to survive and thrive in harsh climates or in poor soil. But I suspect the real answer is that "food" from this tree is brimming with over 90 different nutrients and 46 antioxidants. Add to this the fact that the leaves of this tree are loaded with vitamins and minerals, eight essential amino acids, and are rich in flavanoids – and one begins to understand that Moringa is truly a superfood.

A cancer patient requires a diet high in vitamins, minerals, enzymes, and amino acids – in their most natural, unadulterated form. None of us can sit down and eat five pounds of kale, 4 pounds of Brussels sprouts, 3 pounds of spinach, etc. But it is possible to get similar nutritional value from organic supplements like "Cruciferous Complete" from Standard Process and products like Moringa.

Moringa contains four times the vitamin A found in carrots; seven times the vitamin C of oranges; over four times the calcium found in milk (milk calcium is not very usable for humans); and twice the potassium that bananas have. You will also find (in their natural, organic form – not fractionated) vitamins D, E, K, B2, B3, and B6 – and the minerals magnesium, manganese, copper, iron, phosphorus, zinc, and selenium in this cornucopia of nutrition.

It's simply no wonder that the leaves and all components of this "horse-radish tree" are anti-tumor, anti-inflammatory, anti-viral, anti-allergenic, and antioxidant – and are the makeup of what is coming to be known as one of nature's most nutritious foods. And the simple advantage of "miracle" foods like Moringa is the fact that they can't hurt you – but have the innate capacity to really help you – particularly if you have cancer. Find information about acquiring this product at www.moringa.com.

IODINE

As a population, we know little about iodine or the wondrous things it can do for us. Instead, we tolerate our bouts of sickness and chronic illnesses with no thought or regard as to why these routinely inhabit our bodies. And, lo and behold, lack of iodine is one of the major culprits.

Many of us are old enough to remember when they used to put iodine in our bread and bakery products. About fifty years ago the average American got approximately 1 mg. of iodine daily in their diet. And guess what? Thyroid problems were rare – as was fibrocystic breast disease and breast cancer. What happened? Through its infinite wisdom, the food industry (driven by the FDA) decided to remove the iodine from bread and bakery items and replace it with bromine. Read this: iodine good – bromine bad. Our country's health has been on the decline ever since. Listen to what Dr. Jim Howenstine, M.D., said in 2005 about this tragedy:

"Forty years ago the food industry decided to remove iodine from baked goods and replace the iodine with bromine. Iodine and bromine appear similar to the thyroid gland and bromine easily binds to the thyroid gland's receptors for iodine. Bromine, however, is of no value to the thyroid gland, unlike iodine, and it *inhibits the activity of iodine in the thyroid gland.* Bromine also can cause impaired thinking and memory, drowsiness, dizziness, and irritability. This substitution of bromine for iodine has resulted in nearly universal deficiency of iodine in the American populace. Iodine therapy helps the body eliminate fluoride, bromine, lead, cadmium, arsenic, aluminum and mercury. Could this substitution of bromine for iodine have been carried out to increase diseases and thus *create more need for pharmaceutical drugs?*"

Now, Doc, that's a very interesting question. Could it? You be the judge.

There is no doubt, however, about the nearly universal deficiency that Dr. Howenstine references. We simply do not have enough iodine coursing through our blood and tissues to help prevent many of the diseases that plague us. I sincerely maintain that, if Americans had blood/tissue sufficiency of both vitamin D3 and organic iodine, most sickness and disease would leave us. This is **so very important to you and your health – that I must repeat it**:

If you and I simply got sufficient (way above governmental RDA's) vitamin D3 and organic iodine into our daily diet, we could eliminate most sickness and disease – especially ***CANCER!***

I realize that you must now be saying, "Bob – have you lost your mind." Well, the answer is "no" (my wife might argue) and the studies prove it. More importantly, outside of the clinical setting are the many lives that have been changed, healed, and saved by bringing their bodies to sufficiency in both iodine and D3.

You could go out and buy a kit to check for iodine deficiency – but my suggestion is to not bother or waste the money. Instead, go to the drug store and acquire a $3 bottle of tincture of iodine. "Paint" a two-inch square of this liquid on the inside of your forearm (it dries and starts to soak in immediately in most) and watch how fast it disappears. If it has vanished in 24 hours or less – you are severely deficient and need to supplement with iodine. If it lasts for 36 hours – you may still be slightly deficient. If the iodine is still readily visible at 48 hours – you are probably sufficient, and you would be one of the few. Don't do this if you are allergic to iodine – very few are. And if you are, you already know it.

Once you have concluded that you are deficient, think about adding a natural, organic iodine to your supplement regimen. I recommend prolamine iodine, made from zein, a protein found in organic corn to which iodine binds. This product can be acquired from Standard Process in 3 milligram tablets for about $11-$12 per bottle. Obviously, I do not know what each individual's health condition is or what drugs they are taking. As a result, I must advise all to consult with their physician before starting an iodine supplementation program. Unless you are allergic, though, it probably cannot hurt you and will only improve your health.

Know, however, that your blood must reach a 1.5 gram or 1,500 mg. level to become iodine sufficient. Many of us will discover that we are very deficient and will require a lengthy course of iodine supplementation. If I found myself to be deficient in iodine and, after determining that I was not allergic and there were no contraindications with drugs (I take none), I would start this program – without question – if I had cancer or, even if I didn't. Iodine is ***absolutely critical for health.*** You must decide for yourself.

CHLORELLA

Dr. Tony O'Donnell, in his fabulous new book *Miracle Heart Health Secrets*, conveys the following regarding chlorella:

> "Japanese researchers report that chlorella algae can raise the level of protein albumin in the blood. Albumin, one of the body's most powerful antioxidants, transports toxins to the liver and moves vitamins, minerals, fatty acids, hormones, and other substances throughout the body."

Chlorella is a single cell algae that is a great source of protein that is easily digested. It is known to contain more than 20 vitamins and minerals and nucleic acids which help cells to regenerate. It is rich in chlorophyll which is one of nature's greatest detoxifiers. This super nutrient will help to get the heavy metals, pesticides, and other poisons out of your system.

Chlorella is an immune system booster and increases the macrophage (eliminates bad stuff from the blood) production in the body. And as Dr. O'Donnell puts it, "Since increasing macrophage production can accelerate destruction of cancer cells and harmful bacteria, chlorella might be particularly beneficial for people suffering from cancer or HIV. Chlorella is used to treat a wide variety of illnesses, including allergies and asthma. It also lowers cholesterol and blood pressure, reduces hardening of the arteries, and helps fight chronic fatigue."

Think about this: The Japanese are heavy smokers and drinkers and live in a highly industrialized country with an abundance of toxic wastes. Yet they have become one of the longest-living groups of people on earth. Chlorella plays a big part in their longevity.

Simply put, chlorella is a true super food. I would not hesitate to include it in my anti-cancer protocol – and neither should you. Give this substance priority consideration, even if you don't have cancer. Make sure to acquire only the "cracked cell" or "broken cell wall" varieties. These types increase the benefits of this food significantly. There are several good ones available. I like "Sun Chlorella®" – but you choose what you think is best.

My friend, Tony O'Donnell, is an Irish-born Naturopath and known as "The Herb Doc." He is an author, T.V. personality, radio host, and was awarded "Man of the Year" by the Leukemia Society in 2001. When it comes to food – and what works for cancer – Tony is the real expert. Besides that, he's one of the nicest guys you will ever meet. Visit Dr. O'Donnell's website at www.radiantgreens.com.

THESE ARE THOSE

The aforementioned supplements feature the baseline additions to the critical cancer diet that I would, without hesitation, include in my daily protocol if I had cancer. As stated, I would partake of many – or most – of them, even if I didn't have cancer, as healthy and immune building preventatives.

There are several other very good supplemental products to which I would give careful consideration. You will find these, with brief descriptions, in Chapter Eight. Onward and upward.

CHAPTER SIX

"STEP THREE OF THE CANCER DIET: RESTRUCTURED, IONIZED WATER COULD SAVE YOUR LIFE"

"Water is life's mater and matrix, mother and medium. There is no life without water."

Albert Szent-Gyorgyi, Hungarian Biochemist
Nobel Prize in Medicine, 1937

RECENTLY, I undertook a serious and in-depth study of water over a period covering approximately four months. I am now much less confused than when I started. Actually, I have now earned my "self-proclaimed" undergraduate degree in H20 and have become truly educated regarding the vital importance of this life-sustaining fluid – especially in its "ionized" form.

Water is an enigma to many – make that most – people. They know they need it, but they don't seem to know why or in what form. I'd like to have a dime for every time I've heard that "water is water." Well, I can assure you that while it may all look the same, it is definitely – and conclusively – *not* all the same. And here's what I mean.

Water out of the tap is not the same as bottled water. Water flowing down a stream from a glacier is different from Mississippi River water. Everglades swamp water differs greatly from that in the Great Salt Lake.

You get the picture. We have difficulty discerning, however, the quality, structure and properties of the water we drink and pay no mind to its purity, hydrating effectiveness, mineral content or electrical characteristics (what's that?). Nor do we seem to know why these elemental attributes are important.

Book after book, study after study, and paper after paper have been produced about water. The Internet is a virtual library on water. While you can continuously study this never-ending volume of H2O paraphernalia, you will probably wind up confused and come to the prevailing (and cop-out) conclusion that "water is water," but you would be missing one of the simplest and most valuable ingredients to good health.

Most of us know that the body is about 70% water, we should drink eight glasses a day, humans can go for weeks without food but only three to four days without water, etc., etc. What we don't know – or fail to realize – is that most water is acidic, much of it is "dead" (no minerals), tap water is full of poisons (chlorine and fluoride), it struggles to hydrate our cells, and contains oxidants rather than antioxidants.

Let's break it down. We've already discussed the importance of the acid/alkaline problem with cancer patients. Most humans are acid, which promotes disease. Remember the pH scale. The letters pH stand for "potential of hydrogen" or "per hydrogen" which just equates to the amount of hydrogen atoms (H+ acidic) and/or hydroxide ions (OH- alkaline) within a substance. So a pH of 8 would mean many times more hydroxide atoms (alkaline) than a pH of 6 (actually, 100 times more). This is important for two reasons. First of all, water with a pH of 8 would have a tendency to alkalinize us while that of 6 would acidify our bodies. Secondly, hydrogen is essential to fuel us and to heal us.

Water has electrical energy that can be measured in millivolts (no, you won't be electrocuted), and that capacity for electrical charge can be positive or negative and lost or gained over time. What is imperative to understand here is that positively charged hydrogen atoms or ions (H+) make water acidic, while a hydrogen atom that bonds with an oxygen atom produces a negatively charged (OH-) molecule of water that is alkaline. The science goes way beyond what we care to pursue, but this is what you need to know.

The positive or negative characteristics of water are called the oxidation reduction potential (ORP) because of their ability to promote or neutralize free radicals in the body. Acid and alkaline are always at war within us and, because we constantly overload our systems with acid food and drinks (the H+ positive hydrogen ions) – acid usually wins and our bodies become acidic over time (read cancer). Conversely, if we concentrate on eating foods and drinking water with negative hydroxyl ions (OH-), we increase the negative charge or negative oxidation reduction potential. These OH- ions then bind to the H+ (acidic) ions to neutralize the free radicals that cause the "rusting" or "rotting" of the human internal terrain.

Increasing the alkalinity leads to decreasing the oxidation. The effects of free radicals or oxidation of the cells can be better described as hepatitis, cirrhosis and cancer in the liver; pancreatitis, diabetes and cancer in the pancreas; and nephritis, nephrosis and cancer in the kidneys. While all are bad, do you see the common denominator to all of these? Yes, it's cancer.

So, ionized water increases our alkalinity and uses its negative oxidation reduction potential (ORP) to neutralize free radicals. There is one more important aspect that can be attributed to negatively charged, reduced water – low microclustering of the water molecules. This is a hot topic. There seems to be somewhat of a split school of thought within the scientific community on this subject. Many researchers believe that water is dynamic and can have no stable, low microcluster capability. An equal number believe the opposite and offer proof through studies using nuclear magnetic resonance testing that show that the electrolysis process reduces clustering of water molecules from 10-20 (or more) per cluster for regular tap water down to 5-6 for ionized water. This process reduces the surface tension of the water and allows for solubility and cell permeability.

And what did my Great Hekawi Grandmother say about the proof being in the pudding? So, I had to put it to the test. Water has a half-life of 5-10 minutes in the stomach depending on how much you drink, how fast, and how cold it is. This means that the water (needing no digestion) has a 50% chance of having left the stomach completely within that period of time. Believe me, for good quality ionized water this is true and, like Elvis, it has left the building (stomach) within that time frame. It works for me and with all users with whom I have spoken. From experience you know that if you guzzle 12-16 ounces of any liquid you can feel it "sloshing" around down there for quite some time. On the other hand – and because of its low microclustering character – you can literally jump on a trampoline 5 minutes after consuming an equal amount of ionized water and feel no discomfort. And that's because it has already been transported out of the stomach and is working its way into the cells. And I've heard that exact story from many who have tried it. There's the empirical or "life" (not clinical) evidence.

Because of its low microclustering capability, its strong alkalinity and, most importantly, the low negative ORP and free radical scavenging capability, *I believe that ionized water is a mandatory, baseline "treatment" for those with cancer*.

Many people ask about distilled and reverse osmosis water. I simply tell them that they are acidic with all (or most of) the nutrients (minerals) removed. Sure, it's pure. But at what cost? Water without minerals will scavenge them from your bones and everywhere else in your body as it moves through you. Water has an inherent need for minerals and, if it doesn't have them, it will go find and take them. The stream running down the mountain picks up minerals from the rocks, earth and sand that it travels over. Don't let it happen to you. Bag the distilled and RO water, the tap water, and bottled water, as well. Almost all water that is sold in a plastic container is acid and was bottled, on average, *one to three years prior to your purchase!* Gee, I wonder where it's been?

Since your body is over 70% water, doesn't it make sense to put the best water possible into it? I think so, especially if you have cancer. And you'll feel the difference.

There are many different machines out there that produce ionized water. I have researched them – and you should too. The technology is pretty much the same across the board with this equipment, with slight differences, but the quality varies widely.

Operation is generally quite simple and the electrolysis process is straightforward. With most machines, after installing a provided splitter on the tap, with the flip of a small lever, water is diverted through a hose and into the machine where it is filtered. The chlorine and contaminants exit here. The water then enters the electrolysis chamber where it passes over, around and between titanium plates that are platinum coated or plated. These serve as the electrodes (electrical conductors). The minerals in the water are "ionized" which, basically, restructures the liquid into its alkaline (OH-) and acid (H+) components. The water then flows out of the machine via two different ports; one for the acid water and one for the alkaline. Fluoride is an acid molecule so it passes out the acid port and down the drain. Since the water molecule is fundamentally "split" at this point, the chambers shunt the lower pH fluid through a smaller hose and the high pH liquid through the main, upper hose. Settings on the equipment (most brands) will allow the user to produce alkaline water to about 10.0 pH and acid water to about 4 or 5 pH. A few go as high as 11.5 pH and as low as 2.5 pH.

But you wouldn't drink 2.5 pH or 11.5 pH water, would you? The answer is normally "no" you wouldn't. It appears that Americans have no fear of consuming 2.5 pH soda pop, however. The equipment that produces these pH extremes does so for specific reasons. Most people don't know that when water gets below about 2.6 pH it kills most bacteria and pathogens known to man. This makes it ideal for open wounds, burns, and infections. In addition, 11.5 pH water is an emulsifier and will remove oils and pesticides from fruits and vegetables. I soak all my produce in 11.5 pH water for 5-10 minutes before storing or eating. When I take them out of this very high alkaline liquid, the water is actually yellow – reflecting the chemicals and pesticides that have been removed. It also will extend the "shelf life" of your produce to at least twice its normal refrigerator existence. And, since its high alkalinity draws out acids, many with arthritis and gout, muscle soreness or tissue injuries, utilize the 11.5 pH water to soak in to "pull out" acids associated with inflammation, injury and pain. Yes, I've seen it work.

Usually, drinkable ionized water falls in the 8.0 – 9.5 pH range. Most who set out on the ionized water journey start at 8.5 and work up to 9.5. This allows for a build up to higher alkalinity in the body that can bring on a "healing process" known as a Herxheimer reaction. It is actually a good thing and demonstrates that the alkaline water is challenging the body's disease-causing acidosis. Depending on the severity of one's sickness or degree of acidity, this "reaction" should be relatively short-lived. Symptoms can be lethargy, tiredness, headaches, slight nausea, etc. If this reaction gets too severe, one should back off of the pH (read reduce) but INCREASE the volume of water ingested. As a result, the body will flush the toxins that have been "stirred up", while reducing (slightly) the pH will slow the stimulation of these internal poisons.

We spoke of the Hunza (or Hunzakut) people in a previous chapter regarding the nitrilosides in their food, namely apricot kernels. The Hunza have one of the longest life spans in the world, routinely living to over 120 years old. Yes, they have a nutrient-rich diet that is devoid of all the crap and processed food that we ingest. But they also drink water from pristine glacial streams. The structure of ionized water is similar to that of "Hunza" water. Dr. Henri Coanda and Dr. Patrick Flanagan (and others) discovered that this glacial water had a very high natural mineral content, a high alkaline pH, and a load of active hydrogen with that very important negative oxidation reduction potential (ORP). Can we make the connection?

The technology that has become alkaline, ionized water was birthed in Russia back in the 1950's. About 36 years ago the Japanese grabbed hold of the technology and perfected it. During the past three and a half decades it has gone through many phases, much research, and endless testing. Restructured ionized water, produced by electrolysis machines, has become a proven and accepted methodology in that country and drinking this substance is a way of life for the Japanese. It should also be so in America but, unfortunately, it's not. As a matter of fact, one Company's line of ionizers is now officially classified and certified as a medical device in Japan. And this is the company that I endorse and, as always, I must tell you that I receive nothing for saying so.

I informed you earlier that I spent about four months investigating both ionized water and the equipment that produces it. Within the past ten minutes, you should have developed a sufficient, working knowledge about this water, its efficacy, and importance for cancer patients. During the course of this water quest, I also reviewed the multitude of companies that produce ionizing equipment and their individual electrolysis technologies and "water reducing" machines. What I discovered is that there is a very wide range of quality and pricing among the many manufacturers. You can literally buy an ionizer for as little as $600 or as much as $6,000. You could also purchase a plastic bottle with a mineral filter that, in my opinion, will not get you anywhere you need to go – as we have previously discussed.

In the field of ionization and electrolysis, it became very evident to me that you really get what you pay for. While there are a few machines that will give you excellent alkaline water and fewer that will provide a relatively high-negative ORP, there are many others that won't do so and most for not very long. You must decide what works for you, what you can afford, and which technology or equipment makes you the most comfortable. Herein, I must advise you, is another "caveat emptor" or buyer beware scenario.

When looking for a water ionizer, please (and I must emphasize this) exercise a great degree of diligence. Most of the equipment in the market-place today simply does not have the power to produce the recommended 9.5 pH drinking water, the 11.5 pH cleaning water (for fruits and veggies), nor the 2.5 pH sanitizing water (killing microbes/bacteria) – even though *they claim to!* The machine you select should have adequate power to microcluster the water and enough "electrolysis" to give a minimum minus 300 milli-volt (preferably much lower) antioxidant level and, most importantly, to maintain a large portion of that negative charge for two to three days. I have to tell you – most machines *cannot do that.*

It is very important to actually see the water "tested" so that you don't get stuck with a machine from a company with a low price tag, great promises, and no results. An electrolysis unit should have enough internal "plate" surface area to provide you with as many gallons per day as you want without breaking down, shutting off or overheating – and it should have enough power from a very reliable transformer to cause efficient and effective electrolysis and a cleaning system to prevent calcium from building up on the plates.

You will hear many ionizers claim to be equally as good as any other – at half the price. Don't you believe it. Most of them will not produce the lasting antioxidants (ORP) nor the quality of water that they claim.

I made my choice based upon quality (actual, not perceived), longevity, and the "studied proof" of its ionized water and overwhelming support from literally thousands of users via their life-changing testimonies. And, no, I didn't just read about these – I have actually talked to the people, heard their stories, and viewed their results first hand. Their experiences were truly life changing.

Do your own homework – get what you feel is best for you. In a moment, I will tell you what I chose. Prior to that, though, let's listen to what some of the experts say about alkaline, ionized water, and their reasons for why you should drink it.

Dr. Ray Kurzweil and Dr. Terry Grossman, authors of, *Fantastic Voyage: Live Long Enough to Live Forever*, state the following:

"Consuming the right type of water is vital to detoxifying the body's acidic waste products and is one of the most powerful health treatments available. We recommend that you drink 8-10 glasses per day of this alkaline water. It is one of the simplest and most powerful things that you can do to combat a wide range of disease processes."

The author of *The pH Miracle*, Dr. Robert Young, says that "to maintain or restore your body's natural pH balance for optimal health, drink restructured, ionized water which is rich in anti-oxidants and alkaline minerals. Ionized water helps reverse the effects of acid accumulation in the body, the root cause of degenerative diseases and aging."

Dr. Gabriel Cousins, author of *Conscious Eating*, says it simply:

"Water ionization could be one of the most important health breakthroughs in our era."

"Alkaline water produced by a water ionizer has become the most important advancement in health care since Sir Alexander Fleming's discovery of penicillin." This quote (and a very stunning one at that) was voiced by *Cancer Cure* author, Dr. William Kelly.

Dr. Theodore Baroody, D.C., N.D., Ph.D. Nutrition, and author of the classic book, *Alkalize or Die*, provides his opinion on this elixir of life:

"After years of very positive continuous clinical experiments that I am conducting with hundreds of clients using electronically restructured, alkaline water, it is my opinion that this technology will change the way in which all health providers and the public will approach their health in the coming years. My suggestion is to drink restructured, alkaline water whenever possible."

The following statements all came from the detoxifynow.com website:

"Ionized water has millions of hydroxyl ions per glass. No other water has this incredible benefit. Hydroxyl ions 'neutralize' cancer causing and destructive free radicals in the body.

"Ionized water is thousands of times more healthful to your body than any other water. And the proof 'is in the pudding' so to speak. Everyone who drinks ionized water, either in its natural state as glacier milk, or from a properly built and functioning water ionizer, lives in a state of health light years beyond those that don't.

"One glass of ionized water can hydrate your body better than gallons of any other water.

"Ionized water alkalizes your body better than the only other method (eating a 100% organic and raw vegetarian diet).

"Cancer, obesity, high blood pressure, diabetes, arthritis, kidney/renal disease, cardio-vascular disease, ad infinitum, are all slowed, stopped, and in most circumstances reversed when drinking ionized water.

"Ionized water can flush toxins and poisons out of your body better and with considerably less negative effects than any other detox program/protocol."

This last statement has been verified in spades by Dr. Hiromi Shinya, the co-developer of the colonoscopy and a life-saving medical tool used for the endoscopic treatment that removes polyps in the colon. His technique for removing these growths, called the "Shinya Method," is widely utilized in colonoscopies today. Dr. Shinya has performed more than 370,000 of these medical tests and over 140,000 polypectomies and is a staunch supporter of ionized water, mainly because he has seen its results in the human colon. The video evidence, both before and after the usage of ionized water, is stunning. You can view these videos yourself by entering the good Doctor's name into your search engine – hopefully, after you're done eating. Dr. Shinya puts all of his patients on a high alkaline diet with a minimum of one gallon of ionized water (depending on body size) per day. All of the cancer patients that he and his team have treated have a ZERO recurrence of ANY kind of cancer. In his book he states flatly that if people would follow his recommended lifestyle – there would be no cancer at all.

If I were looking for an electrolysis unit today, I would choose the SD501 made by the Enagic Company. I have explained most of my reasoning for this decision in earlier comments. The versatile, multi-function SD501 is rather expensive at just under $4,000, but worth every penny and is simply the "Rolls Royce" of water ionizers. Other impressive units from this company range in price from $1,300 (travel) to $6,000 (commercial). The water that they produce is referred to as "Kangen Water™," which is a registered trademark of the Enagic Corporation. No other company's ionized water can legally be called by this name. They were the first, having been in business for over 30 years, and have been the unquestioned leader of this industry since their first unit was built. Most of their equipment will last for yours or my lifetime and, if we outlive it, they will recondition it for a small fee.

The fact is that I only want to buy one ionizer, I want it to be durable, and to always produce the high alkaline, negative ORP, low microclustered water that my body really "thirsts" for. For all of my requirements, including the 2.5 acid water feature and the 11.5 super alkaline water capability, only Enagic fit the bill. Some may disagree with me – that's O.K. Establish your own criteria and find the one that works best for you. Although the Enagic unit is a little pricey, it is more than worth it for what you get – and it might just save your life. Remembering that a single day in the hospital for a cancer patient now far exceeds $6,000, this could be a real bargain. I don't believe mine will ever expire and I plan on living a lot more years. It will still probably outlive me – that's how good I believe it is. And, in fact, it is the only unit that I found to be really worthy (health enhancing) *at any price*.

Whatever your choice, find a way to get good quality, highly alkaline, negative ORP, low microclustered, ionized water into your body as rapidly as you possibly can – especially if you have cancer. Do not drink a lot when you take medications as it makes them more potent. Take only a small amount with your meds and allow 30 minutes or so on either side of this for consuming larger quantities. Also, stop drinking about 20 minutes before you eat and wait for at least an hour after meals to resume.

Checkout the Enagic USA corporate website at www.enagic.com and review the technology and equipment. You can find out how to acquire a water ionizer through this site or by calling their home office in Torrance, California, at 866-261-9500 or 310-542-7700.

If you choose to go another route for ionized water, please research thoroughly and choose wisely. You'll be glad you did. Giddiyup!

I have no financial interest in the Enagic Company nor do I receive any remuneration for my recommendations.

CHAPTER SEVEN

"THE TREATMENTS: WHAT I WOULD DO AND WHY"

"Is DMSO effective as a cancer treatment? YES. In the documented research literature and in actual cases we have witnessed firsthand, evidence shows that it has brought about total remission on many high grade, aggressive tumors which had progressed (metastasized) to the lymph nodes and other areas of the body."

Camelot Cancer Care – Tulsa, Oklahoma

JUST prior to writing this chapter, I got a call from a friend of a young couple whose 4-month-old child was in the hospital with cancer. Actually, the child had not left the hospital since birth, as a large growth was immediately evident on his left side, postpartum. Within two weeks he was diagnosed with a rare form of cancer called Infantile Fibrosarcoma.

While I'm sure the doctors want to save this little boy, the subsequent story of his short life is horrific. He has been subjected to multiple chemo-therapy drugs, transfusions, and CT scans. Physicians have infused him with steroids and other medications. He struggles to breathe and his heart rate has many times raced to over 200. The tumor that is close to his little heart and lungs continues to grow unabated and has eaten through blood vessels causing bleeding into his chest cavity. The chemo causes him to throw up acid since there is no food in his tiny stomach. His heart is now producing PVC's (pre-ventricular contractions), he has partial vocal cord paralysis, he continues to bleed, and the tumor is growing more aggressively.

The friend who called was hopeful that the baby's father would contact me and that I might be of some assistance. I assured him that I would do anything that I could. I do not treat, diagnose, or advise cancer patients. I merely tell them what I would do, based upon their situation, if I was in their shoes. Unfortunately, there is probably nothing that can be done for this poor, baby boy. Based upon my limited knowledge of the case and reading the "on-line" journal and profile, and my comprehension and understanding of conventional cancer treatments and therapies, there is little that anyone can do at this point. And while I hope and pray that he survives and grows up and lives long, I really don't think he will.

Whether or not he would have survived with "alternative" treatments from the start, I cannot say. What I know to be certain, however, is that the barbaric litany of drugs, poisons, tests and therapies that he has been subjected to will probably be his end – not the cancer. It's just the sad and tragic truth. And I so much hope that I am wrong.

What is commonly referred to today as "alternative medicine," is actually as "conventional" as it gets. When did it become "alternative" to treat yourself with the elements that were designed to heal you in the first place? When did we begin to disregard the human immune system as the primary disease fighting mechanism and give that title over to anti-biotics, antacids, poisons, and radiation? Why have we become so intellectually challenged when it comes to treating the diseases that ravage our bodies and doing what is right and necessary to save our own lives?

Don't you see? These man-made ideas of health and healing are the true unconventional protocols – the real "alternative medicine." And as long as we subscribe to this pseudo healing status quo, we will continue, as a people, to physically deteriorate, suffer, and die prematurely.

The main problem relating to helping this little boy is that the parents would not be able to get him out of the hospital and treat him with anything that was not accepted by the FDA and the AMA – even if they wanted to. They would be stopped. They would simply not be allowed to do it. We've all heard the stories about children who were "forced" to undergo chemotherapy and the "unconventional" conventional treatments – even against their will and that of the parents. In some cases, parents have been arrested (and children taken away) for not adhering to the requirements and will of allopathic medicine (see the following site for 2 examples: www.lewrockwell.com/sardi/sardi110.html). Friends, when and where does this madness stop? When do we stop getting "treated to death?"

This little boy is just one case study – there are literally thousands more. And if he doesn't make it, his death will be classified as unfortunate and the certificate will say that he died of heart failure, stroke, or some other malady – not cancer. That's the way it works and that's how statistics can be "adjusted" to make it look like we're gaining on the "Big C".

When it comes to treatments, obviously I would avoid any that this child has suffered through, again and unless, it was absolutely necessary, in the short term, to save my life. And, in most instances, I believe that anyone with cancer should forgo these – if they have a choice. Having said that, there are specific situations where individual conventional cancer protocols are warranted, but they are very rare, few, and far between.

The purpose of this chapter is to outline and forward natural, therapeutic treatments, falling outside of mainstream procedures, that are making a significant difference in extending the lives of very advanced cancer patients and, some say, healing them. If I had any diagnosed form of cancer, or undiagnosed suspicions, I would seriously consider one or more of the listed therapies.

First of all, however, a little review and some "common sense" directions are offered. Following that theme, please keep in mind how "uncommon" common sense is today. I believe we must follow what is right, not what is convenient or politically correct. The problem is that often we have a difficult time distinguishing which is which. That's the reason that this book is always exhorting you to do your homework and to find the truth. Where cancer is concerned, the truth is virtually the only hope for your survival. Seek it diligently.

In an earlier chapter I advised that cancer patients should have an advocate or coach. When it comes to auxiliary treatments, this is critically important. While some of these can be done at home, it is possible that you may not be able to accomplish them alone, depending on your specific situation and amount of disease. If you must travel to a clinic for outpatient services, you may need assistance with transportation, depending on your condition. Many of these centers have one to three week therapy protocols and you must stay in a hotel or otherwise acquire your own lodging. With an extended stay, you must also be able to maintain the cancer diet, which is very difficult in a restaurant environment. For these reasons, and others, it is critical that an advocate be available to travel with you and/or assist you with implementation and details.

Generally, advocates are either family members or close friends. Coaches, on the other hand, are those familiar with the true and efficacious treatments for cancer and know the requirements and how the process works. And there are not that many out there. They charge a fee (which is ridiculously low) to guide you in what they would do if they were in your situation (like this book does). They do not diagnose or treat cancer. They do not advise you what to do or direct you where to go. They simply offer their expertise, from vast personal experience, on what their plan would be given similar circumstances. I know of a few excellent coaches that I will mention here. I have spoken to each and have studied their protocols – so I know from whence I speak. Their fees range from around $180-$250 or so, and that is all-inclusive from first phone call to when the cancer is resolved. There's not a better deal anywhere. If it were me, I would hire a coach in a heartbeat. They are far more "expert" in the field of cancer than any oncologist of whom I am aware.

Bill Henderson requires that you read his book, *Cancer Free*, prior to procuring his coaching services. Bill is Vice President of the Board of Directors of the Independent Cancer Research Foundation. Sadly, he watched his first wife die of cancer while undergoing only conventional treatments. His anti-cancer regimen has helped literally thousands of stricken cancer patients to heal via alternative protocols. Whether you decide to go with Bill or not, you should get his book and read it. You can also subscribe to his incredibly great newsletter (absolutely free). Get all this info at www.beating-cancer-gently.com/coaching.html.

Burton Goldberg has spent the last 33 years researching treatments for cancer and other diseases. He has produced a DVD entitled "Cancer Conquest: The Best of Conventional and Alternative Medicine" and was interviewed by Suzanne Somers in her new book, *Knockout*. Burton is a wealth of knowledge, a world-renowned cancer expert, and is going strong at over 80 years of age. You can reach him and purchase his consultation services at www.burtongoldberg.com.

I met with Mike Vrentas in his home a short while ago as Webster Kehr (The Cancer Tutor) and I dropped in to see what was new in "electro-medicine" for cancer patients. Of course, Mike makes no claims for any equipment, treatments, or supplements but knows that they have a place in strengthening the immune system and destroying pathogens in the body. He sits on the Board of Directors of the Independent Cancer Research Foundation and has a unique understanding of what cancer is and what is effective in its treatment. You can reach Mike through his website www.cellectbudwig.com (listen to the video that he produced) or email at michaelvrentas@yahoo.com.

Think about getting yourself a coach. It could make the difference for you.

I couldn't leave the coaching arena without mentioning the website of Webster Kehr, The Cancer Tutor. Probably one of the most knowledge-able individuals on the true cause(s) of cancer and the most relentless pursuer of its cure, Webster has compiled a library of data on cancer and its "alternative" treatments – superior to any other site I have come across. I highly recommend you visit at www.cancertutor.com. Plan to stay for a few weeks.

Unfortunately, he is so busy that he lacks time to be a coach. He would be a superb one.

The last area of information that you should consider (that I will include), prior to seeking out additional cancer treatments, involves the subject of root canals. I can hear you now – what the....? Root canals? What does that have to do with cancer? Plenty, it seems.

According to research done by Dr. Boyd Haley at the University of Kentucky, 75% of root canalled teeth have residual bacterial infections remaining in the dentinal tubules. These lingering infections produce toxic wastes that enter the blood stream and can affect any part of the body. And then there's this (and it should give you significant concern): Dr. Thomas Rau, of the Paracelsus Clinic in Switzerland, recently checked the records of the last 150 breast cancer patients treated in his clinic. Now, pay close attention – especially if you are a woman. He found that 147 of them (that's 98%) had one or more root canal teeth on the same acupunc-ture meridian (energy channel) as the original breast cancer tumor! Coincidence? I don't think so – and neither do most of the "alternative" doctors, researchers, coaches, and practitioners who are helping cancer patients to resolve their illnesses. I know, it sounds so "far out" that it is hard to conceive, let alone, believe.

I recommend, however, that you check this out. And I make this recommendation based upon the vast research and study that has been done on this subject, and a visual experience that I had recently. I was presented with a thermograph (produced by a thermogram or digital infrared imaging) of a woman with breast cancer. It was astonishing. A thermogram detects heat within the body that is a result of anomalies, inflammation, or disease. In this particular image, it was evident that there was a definite "trail" from the root canalled teeth all the way to the infected breast! Little doubt was left that the infection had established a route and was involved with the cancerous tissue. Skeptics will laugh at this suggestion and mainstream medicine may have a good chuckle. Don't you, however – you can't afford it.

Do look into this – man or woman. There is too much scientific research and evidence here to ignore it. Get the whole story by visiting www.newhopetechnologies.com/oralconnection.htm.

On to the treatments. If I were a late Stage III or Stage IV cancer patient, I would seriously consider the following treatments. Some can be performed at home; for others you must go to a reputable, anti-cancer clinic. For these types of therapies, a known and approved clinic will be recommended later in this chapter.

COFFEE ENEMAS

As promised, I deliver to you now the feared and dreaded coffee enema! Really, though, it is not hard to do and generally will not cause you any great deal of pain, anguish, or gnashing of teeth. Upon completion (this will be a daily ritual for most), you will feel both relieved and de-stressed and will also have done a great service for your liver. Remember, if you have cancer, the liver (to at least some extent) is always involved. It is your major detox organ and its quality of function, in most cancer cases, has been slightly to seriously impaired.

Coffee enemas have been around for a long, long time – these are not new age liver flushes. Here is a brief description of the process from the S. A. Wilsons website:

"The coffee enema has been used for many years to detoxify the liver. It is a low-volume enema that remains only in the sigmoid colon. There is a duct between the sigmoid colon and the liver called the entero-hepatic circulation system. When the stool reaches this point, it contains many toxins, which are sent to the liver for detoxification. The coffee enema will increase the transit time in the bowel. The caffeine that is absorbed into the entero-hepatic system causes the liver ducts, including the bile ducts, to empty into the sigmoid colon and be eliminated. Releasing the toxins in the liver ducts makes room for toxins from the body to enter the liver for detoxification. The alkaloids in the caffeine stimulate the production of glutathione-S-transferase, which is an enzyme that facilitates the liver detoxification pathways.

"Coffee enemas will not waste minerals and electrolytes because they have already been absorbed in the previous sections of the intestines. The coffee enema is safe, even for people who are sensitive to caffeine, because the coffee remains in the sigmoid colon, where it will not be absorbed, provided the proper amount is used and the enema bag is not placed too high."

Well, there you have it. You can find the complete instructions on the above site at www.sawilsons.com/coffee_enema.htm. You can also procure organic "enema" coffee produced precisely for this procedure at this web address.

Please note that the coffee enema will not only stimulate liver detoxification but also will assist in cleansing the colon. We talked about detox in an earlier chapter and how important it is to all people, especially cancer patients. A great source for all body and organ detoxification processes, their explanations and procedures, is available through a free ebook at the following address:

www.drkelley.com/CANLIVER55.html

Look especially at Chapter IV. This is a great resource. Ladies and gentleman, that's the straight poop.

ULTRAVIOLET BLOOD IRRADIATION (UVBI)

Ultraviolet blood irradiation (UVBI), also called photoluminescence, is a sterilizing procedure that proved its effectiveness at destroying bacteria, viruses, and other pathogens, in the 1920's-1940's until it was literally "pushed" out of the way by the less effective but more profitable antibiotic therapies.

It is amazing to go back, look at the literature, and read the documentation illustrating how UVBI inactivated toxins and viruses, killed all bacteria, increased and activated oxygen in the blood, activated the production of vitamin D, normalized white cell counts, and increased red blood cells, etc. Why on earth is this proven treatment not widely used today?

Dr. Robert Jay Rowen has an excellent white paper that appeared in Volume 14(2), pages 115-132, of the 1996, *International Journal of Biosocial Medical Research*, on UVBI that is subtitled, *The Cure that Time Forgot*. In it he outlines a report from Robert Olney, produced in 1967, in which Olney theorizes that cancer was a result of blocked oxidation within the cells (a view that many hold to be true today). According to Dr. Rowen's paper, "Utilizing detoxification techniques, dietary changes, nutritional supplements, the Koch catalyst, and ultraviolet blood irradiation, he (Olney) reported the reversal of generalized malignant melanoma, a breast cancer penetrating the chest wall and lung, highly metastatic colon cancer, thyroid cancer, and uterine cancer."

It is also interesting to note that UVBI has received FDA approval for its use in cutaneous T-cell lymphoma. Because of that, it is being used "off-label" by alternative physicians for other conditions, as well. Outside of the FDA approval for lymphoma, it is considered legal by most practitioners from the standpoint of long and continuous use (over 50 years) by physicians in the U.S. as a commercially viable product before the present FDA was even in existence (grandfathered?).

Dr. William Campbell Douglass studied UVBI extensively and was so enamored with it and its proven efficacy that he wrote a book about this therapy entitled, *Into the Light*.

Here's how it is done. A small amount of blood is withdrawn, it is passed through a chamber (within a special piece of equipment) where it is subjected to a specific spectrum of ultraviolet light (the same wavelength as light from the sun), and then it is returned to the body. Sounds simple – and it is. This process begins the chain of events (and results) previously mentioned. Several treatments are generally recommended and they are perfectly safe and very effective. If I had cancer, this would be a primary treatment for me. Clinics and contacts for this protocol will be covered at the end of this chapter.

SODIUM CHLORITE (MMS) AND DMSO

First, a little background on both sodium chlorite (miracle mineral supplement or solution) and DMSO (dimethyl sulfoxide). From the www.health-science-spirit.com website:

"Acidified sodium chlorite (becomes chlorine dioxide after activation) is being used in many countries, including Australia and the USA, as an antimicrobial treatment in the food industry, for water purification, and for sterilizing hospital and clinic rooms and equipment. In hospitals it has been used as a disinfectant for a hundred years and in the US meat industry for about 50 years. Health-conscious countries and municipalities are increasingly replacing the health-damaging chlorine with the harmless chlorine dioxide for treating public water supplies.

"In solution, sodium chlorite (NaClO2) is very alkaline and stable but when acidified (activated) it forms the gas chlorine dioxide (ClO2), which smells the same as chlorine, and probably is the strongest all-around antimicrobial and parasite remedy. While it destroys all anaerobic microbes and parasites, it does not damage the beneficial lactobacteria of our intestinal flora. The only residue left in water, food, or in the body after treatment with MMS (miracle mineral solution) is a small amount of table salt or sodium chloride (NaCl)."

DMSO is a by-product of the wood industry and has been used as a commercial solvent since at least 1953. Over 11,000 articles heralding its medical healing properties have been written and 125 countries allow their doctors to prescribe it for many different conditions including pain, inflammation, scleroderma, interstitial cystitis, and arthritis. Unfortunately, not in the U.S. It is FDA approved only for use as an organ preservative for transplants and for interstitial cystitis. In other words, despite the proof of its healing mechanisms, only a token disease can be legally treated with it.

The history of DMSO is rich and is a valuable case study in how, when something is discovered that will treat or heal people outside of pharmaceuticals, it must be stopped. The kibosh was put on DMSO by the FDA back in 1965 when an Irish woman supposedly died of an allergic reaction after being treated with this substance along with several other drugs. No autopsy was ever done nor was a causal relationship established. This case was reported by Carley W. in the September 9, 1965, edition of the *Wall Street Journal.* And, even though DMSO had never been known to harm anyone, the press ran with it and blamed her death on this wonder solvent. It has been suppressed ever since.

The truth is that DMSO is an amazing anti-inflammatory, it reduces and alleviates pain (in many cases almost instantly), it is an anti-oxidant that scavenges free radicals, and many say that it cures cancer all by itself. While there is no clinical proof to support that last statement, I don't doubt its possibility – and probability. The only downside to this substance is its odor, which has been said to be like a "smoky garlic" or reasonable facsimile thereof. Don't be concerned.

There are two different protocols that draw the chlorine dioxide and DMSO together that are important for cancer patients (internal and transdermal). They work synergistically (together) because DMSO has an affinity for neoplasms (cancerous cells) and the ability to get to them and open them up so that the chlorine dioxide will stroll in and kill the microbe inside the cell. As a result, the cancerous cell effectively "reverts" to being a normal cell. This is more than a theory.

It works like this: The two different substances are taken twice daily (morning/evening) about 15 minutes apart. For the internal version, first take 2 teaspoons of DMSO followed a quarter of an hour later by drops of the activated sodium chlorite (not "chloride" – this is not table salt) which becomes the chlorine dioxide. I say "drops" because you must start slowly – say one drop in at least 4 ounces of non-chlorinated water – and work up to 15 drops as your stomach will handle it. Too many drops too fast will make you nauseous.

The transdermal (through the skin) protocol is similar and should be utilized only if there are initial problems with internal ingestion or one wishes to graduate from one to the other. I recommend that you view and follow the entire regimen as outlined on the following site:

www.new-cancer-treatments.org/Cancer/DMSO_CD.html

You can link from the above to a site where you can acquire quality DMSO and the MMS (they are not expensive).

This is really an outstanding treatment. I just learned several weeks ago of a gentleman who had resolved his esophageal cancer utilizing this therapy alone. When you look at the science and healing history behind the two substances involved, once again – as you will hear so often in this book – it makes perfect sense. Many clinics utilize DMSO and introduce it intravenously with other natural substances – like vitamin B-17 (amygdalin/Laetrile). With absolutely nothing to lose, much to gain, and no significant side effects, if I had cancer, this is a treatment that I would definitely do.

RIFE TECHNOLOGY

The story of Royal Raymond Rife is legendary among those who are fighting (and winning) the war on cancer non-allopathically. Here's a brief overview:

Rife was born in 1888 in Nebraska and many years later, as a microbiologist, found himself working for Carl Zeiss in the microscope design and manufacturing business. He ultimately struck out on his own and designed and constructed the "Universal Microscope" with 60,000X magnification that was years ahead of its time. Through an additional technology that he developed, he was able to see live viruses and other pathogens (bacteria, parasites, fungus) in human blood – something that no other equipment or anyone else could do. As a result, the establishment thought it impossible and Rife a heretic. Well, he proved them wrong.

By using the resonance that he discovered to see and identify them, Rife was able to destroy these pathogens by increasing their natural oscillations using radio frequency (RF) energy until he found their mortal oscillatory rate and they distorted and disintegrated. This process did no harm to surrounding tissues.

In 1934, he was given a group of terminal cancer patients to subject to his RF therapy. Within 90 days of treatment, 86.5% had been ***completely cured***. And after adjusting the treatment, the remaining 13.5% were cured within the next 4 weeks (this is a matter of public record). Note, these were late stage, certified, terminal patients. And Rife produced a ***100% cure rate!*** And it's probable that, before beginning this chapter, you had never heard of Royal Raymond Rife.

The U.S.C. Special Medical Research Committee did follow up trials from 1935-37 and verified the results of Rife's 1934 study. Work continued through independent physicians (using Dr. Rife's frequency generators) who successfully treated as many as 40 people per day during the years up to 1940.

But here, unfortunately, is the tragic end to this story. Our benevolent American Medical Association (AMA) stepped up and tried to buy him out with terms that are said to have been outrageous. Rife said "no" – emphatically. At that point, being threatened by a "real" cure for cancer, the AMA went about the business of destroying Mr. Rife. And, knowing they couldn't do it publicly, they began a reign of thievery and thuggery that drove him to his knees and resulted in the theft of all his paperwork and records and the ultimate illegal confiscation of his precious five micro-scopes. He spent the last third of his life in an alcoholic stupor and died at age 83. Go to the following website for an overview of the book on Royal Raymond Rife called, *The Cancer Cure That Worked*, by Barry Lynes:

www.educate-yourself.org/cn/cancercurethatworked1997.shtml

And the following link will lead you to Jeff Rense's great overview of Rife's life, technology, and documentation of his work:

www.rense.com/general31/rife.htm

Believe it or not, Rife technology is available today. Obviously, no one who markets or sells equipment that is purported to do what Royal Raymond Rife did can make any claims whatsoever. That does not belie the fact that it exists. There are actually many, many resonance or frequency devices, claiming Rife technology duplication, available for purchase. The Internet is "rife" with them. It is probable that some of these units are not exactly or precisely what they claim to be. There are a few that are proclaimed by RF and electronics researchers to be very good. When inquiring of the companies that market them, you will receive no data, information, or testimony to the healing efficacy of these devices (to protect the technology and those who sell it from the FDA and the FTC).

Only one that I am aware of, however, has had adequate testing that I would deem appropriate to label it as technology equal to Rife's (there are undoubtedly several others). I have not personally utilized this machine, but have faith in those that have tested and are employing it. I have met with them personally and have seen the equipment and the protocol associated with it. It is the only technology that I am aware of that generates two frequencies – the first being a "carrier" frequency designed to get the second or "main" frequency inside the cancer cells.

This frequency generator is called the GB-4000 and comes with an additional amplifier. It is not hard to operate by following the basic instructions. It is very low amperage so there is no risk associated with it. The website below will give you all the data you need to acquire and utilize this equipment effectively:

www.cancertutor.com/Cancer03/FreqGenerators.html

This site will give you the color-coded, button-by-button protocol for operating the device and will outline the do's and don'ts as this treatment relates to the rest of the anti-cancer therapy. Once you get the hang of it, the rest will be easy. And you will use it often. Understand, however (I must repeat this), that you will get very little information from the manufacturer or seller of this device, simply because they cannot give it to you for fear of being put out of business and thrown in jail. It's hard to believe that this situation still exists in our "medically free" country but, sadly, when it comes to anything that bucks conventional medicine and the pharmaceutical industry, such is the case. The website above will provide you with everything you need to know about this technology and equipment as the site sells nothing so is free to dispense information under the protection of the First Amendment.

The GB-4000 sells for about $2,300 with the amplifier. This may sound like a lot, but it works, can be used by many, and might possibly pay you back with your life. If I had cancer, I would beg or borrow (but not steal) to acquire this unit.

OTHER TREATMENTS – CLINICS

While there are many other treatments that may be considered primary immune boosting and cancer fighting, these just mentioned are the first ones that I would use because they are straightforward, generally simple to administer (at home, with an advocate, or at a clinic), and have shown, in my experience, to be the most effective and beneficial.

There are literally hundreds of "alternative" cancer treatments, supplements, therapies and protocols. Webster Kehr (The Cancer Tutor) believes he has seen at least 500 over the past decade and I have studied hundreds. To be fair, there are good ones and bad ones, effective and ineffective, costly and cheap. You may know of one or be introduced to an idea that "cannot fail and is guaranteed to save your life." Be skeptical, investigate everything, including all that has been mentioned in this book.

Believe me when I say that if you are diagnosed with cancer, two things are *sure* to happen (among others). First, your doctor will tell you that surgery, chemotherapy, and/or radiation are the only way to go to have any chance at all to "recover." Secondly, friends, relatives, well meaning associates and, literally, everyone you've ever known will come out of the woodwork with a "cancer cure" that you must try. Be courteous and thankful, then study and do what you know (by now) to be right. You'll be glad you did.

There are many clinics available for the cancer patient who chooses to utilize non-conventional, non-allopathic measures. Unfortunately, most (but not all) of them are in Mexico, as they are an affront and threat to the American Medical Association and the Pharmaceutical Industry, and have been *driven* out of the country.

There are several other great "alternative" treatment centers in Germany and other areas outside the United States. If I were afflicted with late-stage cancer, I would definitely consider one of these or, particularly, one of the few that I will mention herein. While this is not a complete list and, by no means, declares that these are the only good clinics, these are the facilities that I have investigated and found to be offering protocols that *actually work* for cancer sufferers. You may choose a different one – and that's just fine.

Keep in mind that there are many clinics, cancer care centers, and hospitals now advertising on television – and through other media – that they are employing alternative therapies and "integrative medicine." You now know what the former is – while the latter is surrounded by fog and controversy. In order to "look like" they are supportive of other than conventional treatments that are proving themselves daily, these organizations show the appearance of incorporating natural supplements and certain versions of "alternative" measures to draw customers who are becoming suspicious of allopathic treatments (largely because their friends and family keep dying). So they add a few vitamins here, some dietary advice there, then proclaim it "to be good", and that they are now officially "integrative" and using the absolute "best" of both worlds. Don't you believe it for a second. And don't fall for this – your life may depend upon it. Check it out for yourself.

I have spoken on several occasions with Dr. Robert Rowen who has a clinic in Santa Rosa, California (not named – on purpose) with his wife, Dr. Terri Su. Dr. Rowen is known as the "Father of Medical Freedom" for pioneering the nation's first Medical Freedom Law in the State of Alaska. This law provided statutory protection for alternative physicians. He practices nutritional medicine, chelation therapy (getting the heavy metals and toxins out of the body), oxidation therapy (cancer hates oxygen), homeopathy, herbal medicine, and innovative cancer therapies like ozone therapy, ultraviolet blood irradiation – and others. I highly recommend Dr. Rowen and his clinic. You can reach his staff for information and appointment at 707-578-7787.

Dr. Rowen is also the editor in chief of *Second Opinion Newsletter* (recommended) and has several informative videos on YouTube. Enter his name into your search engine to find them.

Maureen Long is the owner and administrator of Camelot Cancer Care in Tulsa, Oklahoma. I visited with her and toured her clinic recently and came away suitably impressed. Maureen is a passionate woman who utilizes many therapies and protocols (specializing in DMSO) that are safe and effective in boosting the immune systems of cancer patients. She offers a 21-day (can be less or more) outpatient program that is second to none – forwarding many of the protocols mentioned in this book. You will find several testimonies from patients who have been to Camelot in Chapter Ten. Contact Maureen through her website at www.camelotcancercare.com or by phone at 918-493-1011. I would not hesitate to go here with my cancer challenge. And I have full faith that Camelot – and Dr. Rowen's clinic – would be able to assist me in turning my cancer around – although they can't (and won't) make that claim. They are both very affordable with three weeks of treatments costing you far less than 2 days of a conventional hospital stay. Shorter treatment regimens are also available.

The third clinic I would recommend, Magdalena Clinica, has just opened in Cancun, Mexico and is a satellite of the Camelot Cancer Care Center. Camelot is taking advantage of the Mexican constitutional protection of natural healing – which exists under the umbrella of Mayan/Aztec heritage – to offer patients a menu of secure and efficacious immune-boosting treatments which, they believe, are not likely to ever be available within the United States. Camelot could be right about "treatment unavailability" in that last statement, but I hope not. Again, contact Maureen for details. She has outlined to me, in-depth, the therapeutic opportunities at this facility. They are truly incredible and, best of all, they really work for cancer patients. I would not hesitate to vacation in Cancun and get some of the best cancer treatment available in the world.

Camelot and Magdalena are also utilizing a proprietary, special cream formula (botanical based) for breast cancer cases. According to Maureen, "You can actually see the necrotic tumor tissue exuding from the tumors and axillary lymph glands." In addition, they are also employing customized, all natural formulations for patients with two of the more deadly common killer malignancies that mainstream oncology has nothing close to: a specialized spray for squamous cell (oral) cancers and a transdermal cream that they are now using on their prostate cancer cases, with very encouraging preliminary results.

Lastly, and because of great study and long conversations, I would highly recommend the Hope4Cancer Institute in Playas, near Rosarito Beach, in Baja California, Mexico – 30 minutes south of San Diego International Airport. This is an *inpatient* clinic run by Dr. Tony Jimenez and hosts only 4 patients at a time. While slightly more expensive than outpatient clinics, *complete* care is offered – from gourmet vegetarian meals and full medical staff, to several different types of "proven" anti-cancer treatments. At the time of this writing, Hope4Cancer has purchased the building next to it and is remodeling to add six more patient suites and many more treatment rooms. It appears that their great success in assisting cancer patients has demanded more space!

Dr. "Tony," as he is affectionately called, is a "hands-on" physician who, simply put, will take care of you. I met Doc Tony at a conference in Los Angeles and it can truly be said that he is a genuinely nice guy and a compassionate servant of cancer patients. He offers Sono-Photo Dynamic Therapy (using sound and light after ingesting a "sensitizer"), alkalinizing therapies, an exclusive Rapha-EL cancer vaccine, vitamin C, Poly-MVA and Laetrile IV's, whole body and local hyperthermia (soundwave, NOT microwave) – among many other treatments. Hope4Cancer is the only clinic in this area that uses all natural treatments exclusively. Contact Marla Manhart, Patient Liaison, and she will get you brochures and additional information. If you are someone who is deeply afflicted with cancer and really needs total care, I would highly recommend this clinic. Investigate it – I would. You can email Marla at marla@hope4cancer.com and reach the website at www.hope4cancer.com.

For those in the California/Nevada area, I would consider the Century Wellness Clinic in Reno, Nevada, and its great physician, Dr. James Forsythe, who is doing outstanding work with cancer patients utilizing Poly-MVA. In the South, look up Dr. Jimmy Steger at his clinic in Mobile, Alabama. Dr. Steger is a certified nutritionist and Naturopath – the kind of doctor that almost always has the best success with cancer.

As previously mentioned, this is not a complete list of cancer clinics (actually, anti-cancer clinics) nor is it meant to be. I know of these, how they operate, what they forward for treatment, how they do it, and what kind of success they have. I wouldn't recommend them if I didn't. You may find one that you prefer or like better (there are others out there). I would say – good for you. Go for it.

CHAPTER EIGHT

"ADDITIONAL THERAPIES, TREATMENTS, PROTOCOLS AND SUPPLEMENTS – EVALUATED"

"We are talking here about cancer, about an effective treatment called hydrazine sulfate that the government hates – and about the layered lying and outright deception by the government that keeps this drug from the American people."

Health Education Alliance for
Life and Longevity

THE reason that there are so many "alternative" cancer treatments today is that each one of them has made a significant change in someone's life (more likely, many someone's) that has had cancer. After all, who can argue with a healed body?

The common denominator for all of these therapies and supplements – at least the ones that work – seems to be that they are drawn from natural, organic, earth or water-bound mediums or the result of good, non-invasive science (electromedicine, UVBI, etc.). There is no poison in these protocols, no tissue burning or destruction of the body's "good" cells. No, just real food, active water, plant nutrients and extracts, whole, organic vitamin and mineral complexes – just the good stuff.

Herein lies the beauty of "alternative" medicine. There's virtually nothing that can hurt you and so much that can heal you. Nature has given us the tools, but man has chosen to make his own. Beauty and the Beast. Choose wisely, my friends.

Many who are looking for the answer to their cancer have discovered treatments that have yet to be mentioned herein. This does not mean that I believe them to be bad or ineffective, it's simply because some may be application specific (certain situation), and there are many that have not generated enough proof to be considered as "across-the-board" effective therapies. Having forwarded this reasoning, I would like to suggest, in this chapter, some other supplements and protocols that have helped many and led others to cancer freedom. I will also mention one or two mediums that I would not consider and the reasons why.

There will be many left out, undoubtedly, some that somebody, some-where will say cured their cancer. Isn't it truly amazing that there are more than 400 individual alternative applications for cancer out there that have at least some efficacy to treat or heal this disease? Don't you think that this is something that all of our major cancer research institutes should be studying? Shouldn't the billions upon billions of "conventional cancer research" dollars be poured into programs that have a chance of being successful? These should be rhetorical questions – both. Unfortunately, they're not.

Instead, this funding is reserved for the "good 'ol boy" network of traditional research that obtains grant after grant from the National Institutes of Health to do variants of the same old stuff – year after year. Sorry, alternatives are not allowed, not considered, not even on the radar screen. And if the AMA, the FDA, the American Cancer Society and "Big Pharma" have their way, alternatives will be driven from the face of the earth or forced under the wing of the Pharmaceutical Industry to be sold as drugs and drug therapies. We can't allow that to happen.

INSULIN POTENTIATION
THERAPY (IPT)

Back to the treatments. I would not consider Insulin Potentiation Therapy (IPT), simply because it is still a form of chemotherapy. Cancer cells have 10-20 times more insulin receptors than normal cells. IPT is a tumor destruction vehicle that involves shooting a load of insulin into the body followed by, supposedly, "targeted" chemo. The theory is that the cancer cells open their mouths wide because they think sugar is coming and are surprised (and nuked) when the load of poison drops in. Yes, it can and does kill cancer cells. But the same old problems arise. We have to deal with the side effects, and the cancer cells that remain become "super cells" (chemo resistant) and drugs can't kill them. These cells have now become multi-drug resistant (MDR) and they metastasize. As with traditional chemotherapy treatments, IPT fails to address the cause of the cancer and, instead, deals only with the symptoms. Long term, and like most conventional treatments, it generally doesn't work.

If you insist on doing chemotherapy despite the warnings, risks, and eventual failure, IPT would be better than full body poison. I wouldn't do it – but the choice is yours. And if you are one of the fortunate ones whose cancer is said to be in remission or "gone" after chemotherapy in whatever form, don't be fooled into believing that it healed you. It certainly played a part in destroying cancer cells as well as many healthy cells. But, if you are told you are "cancer free" following intensive drug intervention, the fact is that your own immune system somehow recovered enough (or you supported it adequately) to allow you to be where you are *in spite of the chemicals.* Regardless of your new diagnosis of "cancer free," you are not.

Please understand that fact and adopt, if you haven't already, your choice of the anti-cancer protocols within this book to ensure that the malignancy doesn't redevelop.

I could not and would not scold cancer patients for having already undergone what their oncologist or physician advised them to do. There is no merit or righteousness in that. In those cases, it is simply my hope that they remain free of this disease and, ultimately, die of something else after having lived a long and full life.

CESIUM CHLORIDE

I do, however, like and recommend both hydrazine sulfate and cesium chloride as "situation-specific" alternative cancer treatments. They have demonstrated efficacy and provided the baseline to healing for far too many to dismiss them.

Cesium chloride basically raises the pH of cancer cells (makes them alkaline) and does not allow them to feed, thereby, starving the cells. This substance (cesium is the most alkaline of all elements) also neutralizes lactic acid, which is a by-product of cell fermentation. Cancer cells feed by fermenting sugar – producing lactic acid that is then sent to the liver to be reformulated into glucose and, subsequently, returned to feed cancer cells. Cesium chloride stops this cycle. Be mindful that this program must be supplemented with potassium, some swelling may result (could be bad depending on location of tumor), and there is a limit to how much one can take – your body will tell you.

HYDRAZINE SULFATE

Hydrazine sulfate is an inexpensive chemical compound that blocks the conversion of lactic acid back into glucose (like cesium chloride) and also is said to inhibit tumor growth by essentially starving the neoplasm (tumor). The lactic acid cycle, tumor to liver and back, takes a lot of energy that the body can ill-afford to lose when battling cancer. As a result, many patients cycle down into a virtual "pathological anorexia" and quit eating and drinking. This is the cachexic cycle or what is commonly referred to as cachexia (pronounced ke-kex-sia) – or the wasting away associated with the final stages of cancer.

The story of hydrazine sulfate is extraordinary and should be viewed by all considering utilizing this compound. You can find it at www.hydrazinesulfate.org. As with cesium chloride, there is a protocol to follow. Do not take drugs with this treatment and certain foods should be avoided (stay on the cancer diet). You can find complete instructions for both of the preceding products at www.cancertutor.com. Click their titles on the menu at the left side of the home page (thanks again, Webster).

PROTEOLYTIC (PANCREATIC) ENZYMES

In 1906, John Beard postulated that proteolytic (pancreatic) enzymes were the body's main defense against cancer and also useful in its treatment. The story of these "PE's" reads like a novel with sabotage and deception prevalent throughout its pages. This is another case of natural substances knocking heads with conventional medicine. "Alternatives 101" teaches us that when you buck the traditional medical system there will be h.e. double toothpicks to pay. Such is the case with pancreatic enzymes.

Dr. Nicholas Gonzalez picked up the ball from Beard's research and ran with it. And the AMA has been trying to tackle him ever since. Fortunately for you and I (and cancer patients), Dr. Gonzalez is astutely capable of "avoiding the rush" and has a heck of a straight-arm. The Doc appears to be having great success with late stage cancer patients utilizing a protocol that includes diet, aggressive supplementation with nutrients and enzymes, and detoxification (read coffee enemas!).

The anti-cancer effect generated by proteolytic enzymes seems to be due to an immune modulation (activation) that produces a profound anti-neoplastic effect – though the doctors and researchers don't know why.

You can find the history and science behind enzyme therapy at www.dr-gonzalez.com. In addition, although many pancreatic enzyme supplements are available, I recommend Vitalzym. This is a new and improved product available from Energetic Nutrition at www.energeticnutrition.com/vitalzym. I am a firm supporter of pancreatic enzymes and would use them if I had cancer.

HYPERTHERMIA

Hyperthermia (the opposite of hypothermia – brrrr!!) is the process of heating the whole body, the blood, or the tumor itself via different methodologies – some of which, in my opinion, are very suspect.

Tumor-specific hyperthermia involves heating up the tumor to about 108 degrees for 45 to 60 minutes. Radiowave therapy utilizes a probe with radio frequency to heat the cancer cells up to about 150 degrees. Hot baths by total body immersion (only nose and mouth out of the water) at 102 degrees might be very soothing but probably not hot enough to kill any cancer cells, although possible. Most research shows that these malignant cells start to die off when subjected to heat above about 106 degrees.

Hyperthermia perfusion involves a "warmed or heated drug solution" (no thanks) and extracorporeal whole body hyperthermia is done under general anesthesia by heating blood via an extracorporeal loop, usually through the femoral artery, then returning it to the body (think dialysis machine). Radiant hyperthermia is performed using mostly hot water blankets or a thermal chamber.

I believe the jury is still out on the best way to perform this procedure – although it is proven that heat will kill cancer cells. Conventional hospitals like to advertise it but use it exclusively with chemotherapy, radiation and drugs. I wouldn't touch that with the proverbial ten-foot pole.

One of the best locations on the Internet for anti-cancer information is the AlkalizeForHealth website. They have a good page on hyperthermia that you can peruse at the following address:

www.alkalizeforhealth.net/therapeuticbaths.htm.

Many "alternative" clinics utilize various effective methods of this treatment. I would put my faith in these professionals, as the establishments that practice this therapy have a far better understanding of how and why hyperthermia works – and what makes it consequential for cancer patients. That's what I would do.

COLEY'S TOXINS

Coley's Toxins, now commonly referred to as "Mixed Bacterial Vaccine" (MBV), is a form of fever therapy. Understanding that fever appeared to kill cancer cells, William Coley first pioneered the use of this concoction that bears his name in the late 1800's by combining the killed bacteria of streptococcus pyogenes and serratia marcescens (big words for bad stuff) to produce a high fever in cancer patients. The idea was (and is) that the infection would produce an immune system response to destroy the cancer. Guess what? It worked.

"In the West Indies, natives afflicted with syphilis or cancer cured themselves by deliberately subjecting themselves to infection from such high fever diseases as malaria, typhus fever or typhoid fever." Thanks, again, to the alkalizeforhealth.com website for that info. There's that old school, backcountry medicine again. Darned if it doesn't always seem to work. My Great Hekawi Grandmother would be proud.

I would definitely consider Coley's Toxins as administered by a qualified, alternative cancer care clinic. The science is pure and the results are documented. The clinics mentioned in this book (and others) are providers of this treatment.

ESSIAC TEA

You would think that Essiac Tea was poison the way that it is attacked and discredited by mainstream medicine. I believe otherwise.

Essiac was "outed" by Rene Caisse (pronounced Reen Case) via Ojibway natives in the early to mid 1920's. Upon seeing a tribe member heal an English woman's breast cancer with the four-herb compound, this Canadian nurse started on a crusade to treat cancer patients – most of the time for free – for two and a half decades. The healing stories are the stuff of legend. Essiac (Caisse spelled backwards) is composed of sheep sorrel (the backbone of the recipe), burdock root, slippery elm bark, and rhubarb root, and is generally made into a tea. Its method of biological activity is said to be in its ability to jump-start the immune system and normalize the pancreas. It makes sense, then, that it appears to work very well with diabetics in addition to cancer patients.

The American Cancer Society states on their website that "available scientific evidence does not support its use for the treatment of cancer in humans." They seem to immediately refute that when they acknowledge, "there have been many testimonials." They then summarize their editorial on Essiac with the following: "Relying on this type of treatment alone and avoiding or delaying conventional medical care may have serious health consequences." Finally, we agree on something. Indeed, avoiding or delaying conventional medical care *could definitely* have serious health consequences – you'll probably survive! Now, that's serious.

I would not, however, rely on Essiac alone to effect the changes in my body that would defeat cancer. I don't hesitate to say that even though there is a large stack of testimonial evidence to the contrary (that Essiac Tea has healed many a cancer by itself). The cancer diet, ionized water, sunlight, organic supplements, the right treatments and therapies – plus Essiac – yes, that I would do.

Women who are pregnant or nursing should avoid Essiac as well as those with kidney disease, ulcers or colitis (use ionized water), or with tumors where swelling could be a problem. I would use only the original formula or make it myself from organic ingredients. Acquire it from Essiac Canada International at www.essiac-resperin.com or (888) 900-2299. You can learn to make it yourself by watching a YouTube video at this address: www.youtube.com/watch?v=XacqG7isA_E.

KM

KM is in this mix for a very special reason. I discovered this golden elixir (actually dark brown) at a health fair associated with one of the greatest road races in America, the annual "Bloomsday" run in Spokane, Washington. This run generally hosts over 45,000 runners and walkers who stroll through the Convention Center the day before the event to shop the many vendors who are hawking their wares. That's where, in 1988, I was "hooked" by a small man holding a white plastic bottle, printed in orange, "that was gonna change my life." Yeah, right. I've heard that one before. But, you know, he was right. I stepped into the world of KM and never looked back (thanks, Stark!).

Up until a few years ago, KM was the only supplement that I could truthfully say had ever done anything noticeable for me. But I'm getting ahead of myself. First, you need to know what it is besides a brown liquid.

Manufactured by Univera, formerly Matol Botanical, KM is a blend of 14 herbs in a proprietary extract that is very high in potassium and minerals. It is said (on many websites I have visited) to be "the largest selling nutritional product in the USA." KM is advertised to increase energy, purify blood, remove toxins, oxygenate the blood, and improve circulation – among other things. I can attest, personally, that it does these things. After beginning to gulp an ounce or two per day, I was never sick, had no colds or flu, had increased energy and stamina, and knew that my blood was more oxygenated through increased endurance while running and hiking in the mountains. There was no doubt that it was the KM that was making the difference. I attended a seminar in 1990 where I heard a doctor say that if you have been taking KM for at least a year, you would never get cancer. Many agreed. At that same function I talked to an 80+

year old man who had had skin cancer on his nose. He said he just poured the KM down his throat and over his proboscis and the cancer vanished.

I'm not going to tell you that KM will heal your cancer and neither will Univera. But many would testify that they believe it has for them. Whatever the case, I consider it to be an excellent super supplement for cancer patients and I would definitely put it in my arsenal if I had cancer – or even if I didn't. You can find the product by contacting a Univera Distributor on the Internet or through the phone book.

GRAVIOLA – PAW PAW

The fruit and twigs of the graviola and paw paw trees are known by many to have anti-cancer compounds. The graviola tree is native to South America while the paw paw resides in North America. While these are generally thought to be relatively new in the marketplace, much research and many studies have been carried out involving these two natural products.

Both extracts are said to work by blocking the ATP production in the cancerous cells and causing them to "self destruct." They are also known to support the immune system. Most experts involved in plant extract research will tell you that paw paw is 40 - 50% more powerful and effective than graviola. And the Health Sciences Institute, in their January, 2001, *Member's Alert*, stated that graviola was "10,000 times stronger in killing colon cancer than Adriamycin, a commonly used chemotherapeutic drug." Also stated in this article by HSI was that testing had shown that graviola "effectively targets and kills malignant cells in 12 different types of cancer." There is also adequate proof through clinical research done by the National Cancer Institute (graviola) as far back as 1976, and through ongoing studies by Dr. Jerry McLaughlin (paw paw) over many years. Both of these substances have a very long history of use as herbal medicines.

The studies, research, clinical evidence, and testimonies are available for all to peruse at the following sites:

www.pawpawresearch.com

www.graviola.org

You will also be able to locate the best and purest products and the proper methods for using them at these sites (or links therein).

Would I use one of these if I had cancer? You bet.

SUPER JUICES

The "real" super juices are the ones you make yourself from fresh, organic fruits and vegetables (veggies on the cancer diet). However, there are a couple of commercial brands that warrant taking a look at.

Mangosteen juice is full of xanthones, which have proven in many studies to be anti-tumor, anti-fungal, anti-bacterial, and to kill cancer cells. I would consider this juice as a supplement to a good anti-cancer protocol. I believe Xango™ to be the absolute premium mangosteen product in the marketplace – and I drink it. This brand is the only one I could find (from mangosteen) that utilizes the entire fruit (very important). Mangosteen typically is loaded with phytonutrients, particularly xanthones, catechins, flavonoids, and proanthocyanidins. Of considerable importance, however, are the xanthones – as they appear to be the most biologically active components of this fruit. And they are most dense or concentrated in the rind or "pericarp" of mangosteen. That's why it is important for the whole fruit to be used in the supplement – just like Xango™ employs it.

Regarding mangosteen juice, Xango™ was the first – and I believe them to be the best – by far. While no one can say that this product will cure cancer, I have heard some amazing testimonies regarding that exact subject. Certainly, if I had cancer I would be drinking this great tasting supplement. It is one exception I would make to not eating most fruits on the cancer diet. And, please keep in mind, most sickness and disease is caused by – and accompanied by – inflammation. I believe the mangosteen fruit to be one of the greatest natural anti-inflammatories ever discovered. And I sincerely think that this property is bottled exquisitely in Xango™ juice.

Limu Juice may well be the king of the super juices. It is made from fucoidan, which is found primarily in a brown sea plant called limu moui. Fucoidan, also found in many types of seaweed, is loaded with over 70 essential nutrients and has proven, in over 800 independent studies over the last 40 years, to be anti-cancer. A dozen medical journals have reported on this natural extract and its ability to cause cancer cells to self-destruct. I would definitely drink this juice if I had cancer. I have spoken to an anti-cancer expert who believes that Limu Juice is a stand-alone cancer treatment. He has testimonies to prove it. You can scan the Internet for suppliers and the hundreds of studies done that prove the efficacy of fucoidan.

Although it cannot be classified as a juice, a very, very promising "juice-like" nutritional supplement has recently entered the marketplace and appears to be having dramatic results *at the cellular level*. ASEA is said to utilize a patented method for creating and stabilizing molecules native to the human body which provides a pathway to deliver critical "reactive molecules" – molecules that are deemed necessary for maximum cellular health.

I know, you are asking what all that means. Here it is in layman's terms (I had to condense it down so I could understand it):

Through it's "Redox Signaling" – as this process above is defined and known, ASEA boosts the efficiency and effectivity of the body's super anti-oxidants, superoxide dismutase (SOD) and glutathione, by as much as 500%. A recent study also demonstrated that ASEA will increase the uptake of antioxidants while minimizing inflammation. All of this is good news for cancer patients and the human immune system.

Bottom line: Will it heal cancer? I can't say that. Will it give a vastly increased energy and healing capacity to the stricken patient? I don't believe there is any doubt about that. Although ASEA is a relatively new product, the testimonies are starting to come in and are both inspirational and, based upon the science, very credible. And, the really great news is that many of these are related to cancer. Healthy or not; cancer or no cancer; I would seriously investigate this new supplement.

OTHER TREATMENTS/CENTERS

I have the highest regard for the Gerson Institute and the "Gerson Therapy." This therapy was developed by Max Gerson in the early 1900's and is carried on today by his daughter, Charlotte, who has celebrated her 88th birthday. This natural treatment protocol uses organic foods, juicing, coffee enemas, detoxification, and natural supplements as a means to restore and strengthen the immune system and allow the body to heal itself. They are located in San Diego and have a clinic in Tijuana. Contact them at their website, www.gerson.org, to get all appropriate info.

The Whitaker Wellness Institute is located in Newport Beach, California, and is operated by one of the foremost promoters of alternative treatments and therapies, Dr. Julian Whitaker. Dr. Whitaker and his staff have treated over 40,000 patients since 1979, and continue to provide programs that help patients with many different challenges – including cancer. I also give this clinic my highest recommendation. You can contact the Institute at www.whitakerwellness.com.

Dr. Lorraine Day healed herself of a severe case of cancer and rebuilt her immune system through only natural therapies. Her story is incredible and you can actually see pictures of her enormous tumor on her website. This doctor is living proof of the power of diet, nutrition, and faith to heal disease. Dr. Day has developed a complete 10-step program that is likely worth its weight in gold if you have cancer. Another very high recommendation is given here. View her data, information, and acquire her protocol at www.drday.com.

Steve and Suzanne Day operate a wonderful retreat off the beaten path in Stanton, Kentucky, that provides what they call "a quiet place where health is restored." The "Home For Health" specializes in lifestyle-emersion and focuses on (and serves) quality living foods, detoxification, and faith. Participants (patients) receive hands-on training in juicing and food preparation and instructions in nutrition and health (most important for cancer sufferers). I recommend this healing retreat for those with non-late stage cancer. Contact Steve and Suzanne through their website at www. homeforhealth.net.

Normally, I try not to promote any specific company but, sometimes, cannot avoid it because their products or protocols are unique. Additionally, I am not a huge fan of soy foods because the jury is split on their effectiveness and "cancer causing or cancer curing" properties. I have become a genuine supporter, however, of one line of soy-based products – produced by the "Reliv™ International" Company – that is doing amazing things for sick people – especially cancer sufferers. Let me be perfectly clear. I have no stake in this company, financially or otherwise. After extensive research on their product line, the evidence showed that the nutrient-dense food supplements that they formulate are packed with synergistic vitamins, minerals, enzymes and other quality ingredients that are bioavailable and nutritious (remember the cancer diet?). But I needed more proof.

So I spoke with several former cancer patients who firmly believe that these natural food creations saved their lives. They don't and won't specifically say that Reliv™ products cured their cancers. They just know that they are healed. I have also seen volumes of written testimonies on the positive effects that these patented "foods" seem to have on the sick and diseased – once again, especially cancer patients.

I also went back to the research to find out what scientists are discovering about the efficacy of soy as it relates to cancer. Coupled with the obvious and overwhelming success of these products through the volumes of testimonial evidence of strengthened immune systems (which good, organic, nutritious food does for people) and this recent research documenting the phytochemical activity of soy vs. cancer – it made perfect sense why so many thousands of people think so highly of Reliv™ products.

I looked at several studies – but cannot print them all here. I consider the results to be very compelling and, because of what I have physically seen and heard (first hand) from Reliv™ users, know the facts they espouse to be true. Here's a brief summary of several studies from the July, 2010, edition of *Life Extension Magazine* that have been published in respected American Journals from 1998 to the present:

> "Soy derivatives, particularly soy proteins and the isoflavones, exert powerfully beneficial effects across multiple systems of the body. Despite popular misconception at the hands of a vocal group of detractors, soy protein's action on estrogen receptors gives them unique capabilities not found in drugs or other natural compounds. By preferentially acting upon estrogen receptors associated with cancer <u>suppression</u>, soy isoflavones can *reduce* cancer risk."

Whatever your thoughts about soy, I know with certainty that the above concept applies – with no doubt – to Reliv™ products. And until you've looked into the eyes of a healed cancer patient or heard the impassioned testimonies of those who "know" that this nutrition (making no claims) has made an undeniable difference in their lives (they're still on this side of the grass), don't you dare tell me that it can't be so. I've seen it, I've heard it, I know it – it's true. And let the story and debate end there.

I recommend these supplements highly. Can I tell you they will heal your cancer? In a word – no. Can I say that they will work in your body to build your immune system and support the internal functions necessary for healing? Absolutely. You be the judge. Contact is www.reliv.com.

I've seen many cancer patients drinking soda pop – both regular (sugared) and diet. I refer to it as **cancer in a can**. Most of these people are old enough to make their own decisions – good or bad – concerning what they put in their mouths. Unfortunately, our kids are not. They literally drink gallons of sugared drinks a week. It's a major part of the reason why they are overweight, pre-diabetic, lethargic, and have attention deficit disorder – and also why many of them will get cancer. Enter the alternative.

There is an emerging company called Yoli™ that offers what they call their "blast cap" technology, producing nutritious drinks that taste like they are sweetened but contain no sugar. These beverages are loaded with vitamins (live, not synthetic) and minerals and have high ORAC (free radical fighting antioxidants) values. What they don't have is equally impressive. No unnatural flavors or colors, no sugar or artificial sweeteners (only stevia), no preservatives, and no toxic stimulants. Believe me, Yoli™ is the real deal. I highly recommend their nutritional products as a necessary replacement for any sugared or diet drink (aspartame is Mr. Yuk) for kids and adults and, as a "sweet substitute" – on a limited basis – for cancer patients. Contact for these products is the following site: www.yoli.com.

Last, but not least (by a long shot), is chocolate. I know – I said that cancer patients must not eat (ordinary) chocolate. I steadfastly stand by that statement for the most obvious of reasons: most chocolate is filled with sugar – and we know that sugar feeds cancer. However, fast-forward to a new product in the marketplace called Xocai™ (pronounced sho-sigh) that is referred to as the "healthy chocolate." Seems like an oxymoron, doesn't it? Actually, natural chocolate (dark, cacao) is very nutritious and high in anti-oxidants and flavonoids. Yes, it's actually good for you! Xocai™ nutrients are preserved through a low heat and cold pressed process. These products have no added colors, artificial flavors, and no preservatives – and only a very small amount of natural sugar. In addition, this healthy chocolate is gluten, lactose, and caffeine free, diabetic friendly, vegetarian, and has no waxes or fillers.

Come, let's discover *real* chocolate the way that it is meant to be – nutritious and healthful – and its potential use and enjoyment for those afflicted with cancer.

In an article published by "nygal" on the cancerdirectory.com website, April 26, 2009, the following is revealed and gives hope to all of us chocolate lovers:

"'The great news is that in addition to being decadent and delicious, moderate amounts of dark chocolate may play a role in cancer prevention,' said Sally Scroggs, M.S., R.D., L.D., health education manager at the University of Texas M.D. Anderson Cancer Center's Cancer Prevention Center.

"Recent research indicates that dark chocolate's chemicals, which act as antioxidants, have been shown to play a role in reducing cancer risks by helping to combat cell damage that can lead to tumor growth. These antioxidants occur naturally in the plant-based cacao bean, the base of all chocolate products. Cacao beans are, in fact, one of the most concentrated natural sources of antioxidants that exist."

And from the April 18th, 2005, *Science Daily*, comes this:

"Researchers from the Lombardi Comprehensive Cancer Center

at Georgetown University have shown how an ingredient found in chocolate seems to exert its anti-cancer properties – findings that might be used one day to design novel cancer treatments. The study, published in the April issue of the journal *Molecular Cancer Therapeutics*, explains how pentameric procyanidin (pentamer), a natural compound found in cocoa, deactivates a number of proteins that likely work in concert to push a cancer cell to continually divide."

When man gets hold of natural foods and "diminishes" them, we commonly get unnatural products that aren't very good for us (or, in fact, are very bad for us) but really taste good and have a tendency to be addictive. Such is the case with milk chocolate, white chocolate, hot chocolate, etc. We love them and these are what we would call "feel good" or "comfort" foods (yes, "foods" is kind of a misnomer here). Unfortunately, man-made chocolates should be avoided and – must be – by cancer patients.

Having said that, I see no harm in including some Xocai™ products (because of their organic and all-natural make-up) in the cancer diet – in small amounts because of the minute amount of natural sugar they include. Also, put this chocolate in your kid's mouths instead of candy bars and bubblegum. Contact for Xocai™ chocolate is www.mxicorp. com.

It is beyond the scope of this book to cover all the known anti-cancer treatments, therapies, supplements and protocols. As natural researchers and scientists head to the fields and forests, they continually discover plants, shrubs, trees and herbs that are instrumental in enabling the human body to overcome many diseases, including cancer.

Our hope continues to be that these discoveries will be able to see the light of day. Your support for alternative and anti-cancer companies, institutes, researchers, and foundations will help secure this vision and topple the ineffective status quo.

CHAPTER NINE

"Synthetic Visualization: What You Believe Can Heal You or Kill You"

"Errors in the choice of attitudes and beliefs we hold are no less devastating than mistakes in medication or surgery."

Neil F. Neimark, M.D.

JANE (real person, not real name) was diagnosed with metastatic cancer last year. She didn't feel that bad, but knew something was wrong when she went in for tests. CT scans revealed the bad news: multiple tumors in multiple places. Most of her major organs were affected and the prognosis, by anyone's measure, was bleak with the accompanying verdict of only a few short months to live.

After the doctor pronounced the death sentence, he forwarded the "we can get you more time with chemotherapy" standard routine. Jane headed for home, depressed, disillusioned, sick, tired, and desperately frightened. Wondering what to do, she sought the counsel of family and friends who offered support and some "non-conventional" ideas. After righting herself and walking down from the gallows, she decided to employ "alternative" therapies, diet, good water, and supplements to fight her disease. She was on the right track. She started to feel better as the healing process began within her.

Then, for supposed verification that the cancer was retreating, Jane visited her doctor again. He proceeded to tell her that she was expediting her demise by entertaining this silly "non-medical" protocol. Her only hope for extended time still lay in chemo. She was verbally chastised for her foolishness. She went home, got her affairs in order, checked herself into Hospice, and died a week later. Unfortunately, Jane's case is not atypical or isolated.

She conceived that the choice she was given was either a slow and agonizing death by drugs or a more imminent demise by doing nothing. Her medically induced conception was that she was "dead" either way. The seed was planted – and she simply gave up.

Jane was told she was going to die, she believed it, and did what she was told. What you believe, what you conceive – especially with cancer – will play a major role in whether or not you recover.

It is really true that what you can visualize or conceive in your life can, and usually does, come true. We have all seen or heard the stories of elderly, long-married couples who have died within days or weeks of each other. And we would be foolish not to believe the explanation that "one could not live without the other" was the primary cause. As human beings, we often have the innate ability to "will" ourselves to produce specific outcomes. No, it doesn't always happen, but what we believe to be true can – and often does – result in predicted outcomes.

Stress, attitude, emotions, feelings – all play into this scenario – especially with cancer. And here is an interesting take on this from Bob Davis, who overcame cancer twice and has worked with and interviewed many cancer patients (from his *How Your Attitude Affects Cancer Treatments* on the www.healthrecipes.com website):

"Hospitals that specialize in alternative cancer treatment can predict who will succeed and who will fail by the attitude that is expressed by the patient. Success requires a strong, optimistic and dedicated attitude. One must be tolerant of inconvenience and some distress. Recognize that things will be different in your life for a while or even for the rest of your life. You may have to give up some favorite things. So what, do you want to survive? I have seen so many complain because they can't have their favorite food. In the words of Dr. Phil McGraw, 'They just don't get it.'

"One person who overcame cancer with an effective diet program said to me: 'I will never go back to the way I lived and ate before.' This is a winning attitude. Patient, strive to be optimistic. Caregiver, encourage the patient. Attitude can determine your success."

Bob, I couldn't have said it better – no one could have. While there are no guarantees, we must play the odds. And the odds are that a good attitude toward the success of your cancer program could be the difference in your healing.

The "cancer attitude" is a definite psychological situation, but it lends itself directly to physical changes within the body that are critical. This attitudinal effect created by stress or depression is proven to be detrimental to healing. A study entitled, "Influence of Psychological Response on Survival in Breast Cancer", done by researchers at Royal Marsden Hospital in Sutton, England, and reported in *The Lancet*, Volume 354, Issue 9187, in 1999, stated that "A study of 578 women with early-stage breast cancer found that those who revealed strong feelings of 'helplessness and hopelessness' were more likely to relapse or die within 5 years than those with low scores in this category."

A similar study on breast cancer included in the January 7, 1998, edition of *The Journal of the National Cancer Institute* and reported by James Michael Howard through Reuters, deals directly with the physical implications of attitude and stress. The quote from this report states:

"The stress of being diagnosed with and treated for breast cancer can affect a woman's immune system. The effects were so clear that they could make a woman susceptible to illness caused by the chemotherapy and radiation treatment that often comes after surgery. The findings lend weight to the age-old beliefs that a person's attitude to cancer can affect their survival and recovery."

Jeff Grabmeier cited the following Ohio State University study in the *Albion Monitor*:

"Breast cancer patients who feel high levels of stress concerning their diagnosis and treatment show evidence of a weakened immune system compared to patients experiencing less stress, a new preliminary study shows.

"Researchers found that the highly stressed women had lower levels of natural killer cells than women who reported less stress. Natural killer cells are one vital weapon making up the immune system. 'Natural killer cells have an extremely important function with regard to cancer because they are capable of detecting and killing cancer cells,' said Barbara Andersen, leader of the research team and professor of psychology, obstetrics and gynecology at Ohio State University. These results, although preliminary, suggest that psychological stress may play a role in how the immune system responds to cancer."

Dr. Leonard Coldwell is, arguably, one of the best Naturopathic doctors in the world. The author of 19 books and creator of the IBMS™ (Instinct Based Medicine ™ System), my friend Dr. "C" has a proven and verifiable 93% success rate with cancer patients who have not undergone "The Big Three."

When it comes to the main causes of cancer, Dr. Coldwell makes no bones about what he believes, has seen, and can prove. We'd all do well to listen carefully to the following:

"So, what causes an acidic body? Or, what puts it in a state of acidosis and a lack of oxygen? The answer is, first and foremost, *stress*! Nothing can make the body acidic faster than stress. Stress shuts down the metabolism so you can't get proper nutrition. Many illnesses stem from nutritional deficiencies which are actually caused by stress – even if the person has the best diet and nutrition in the world.

"Stress truly does affect our health and well-being. Studies have shown that 86% of all illnesses are caused by stress, while a Stanford University study concluded that 95% of all illnesses are stress related! Even if we use the modest 86% figure, this means that only 14% of all illnesses are caused by other factors not related to stress."

Dr. Coldwell weaves this "stress-factor" into our emotional and physical experiences in his book, *The Only Answer to Cancer*, through this missive:

"Whatever happens in our emotional existence happens in our physical body. Cancer can come from just one trapped and isolated emotion, a feeling of having no choice, helplessness and hopelessness. Mind and body are connected, and any repressed feelings such as wanting and deserving love, acceptance, harmony, success, peace, stability, freedom, and a simple sense of joy in life are translated into appropriate biochemical responses in the body.

"Whatever emotions or past traumas you keep to yourself out of fear of being criticized or laughed at actually turn into poisons in the body. But, the main problem is denial. What I mean by this is that, subconsciously, you know that something is really wrong and needs to change but you take no action to correct it. You continually make excuses or ignore it. Of course, not letting go of past traumatic events is another major root cause of cancer. My solution, instead of 15 years of psychotherapy, is to simply get over it and move on!"

Friends, listen to Dr. "C" and eliminate the stress and emotional baggage – as best you can – from your lives.

Often accompanying stress, depression and hopelessness, is fear. In most instances, whether they show it or not, cancer patients are scared to death. The human instinct is to survive, and if not given any hope that this can or will happen, this instinct – driven by fear – is suppressed and the outcome is usually poor. Shamgar Ben-Eliyahu, from the Tel Aviv Department of Psychology, reported the following in *Science Daily*, February 29, 2008:

> "The psychological stressors of surgery deal a blow to the immune system, but this is hardly discussed in the medical community." And here is the important part. He adds, "Ours is among the first studies to show that psychological fear may be no less important than real physiological tissue damage in suppressing immune competence."

Translate this into the cancer experience and one can readily extrapolate that fear is an immune system suppressor having the ability to break the back of any treatment program, conventional or alternative.

This next bit of information may seem a bit harsh to some and is provided, once again, by Bob Davis, from the same source that was quoted earlier. And while I generally agree with him, I believe that there is a little more to the story that must be added. Bob's take on attitude, optimism, and motivation follows:

"I have dealt with many people who had cancer. Those who overcame had optimistic and aggressive attitudes. Those who did not survive were weakly motivated and vacillated regarding what (and how) they would do to fight the cancer. I know that this generalization is unkind and even cruel to those who were weak and fought the best they could to the end. I am not speaking of them. The ones that I reference are those who were reasonably strong who 'decided' that the fight was not worth the effort, or who had no confidence in an alternative program. I saw them die without trying. We have the popular notion that people are entitled to their opinion. If this is true, then we must consider that we are also obligated to receive the consequences of our actions, including those brought about by our attitude."

He continues with an experience that gets to the real heart of his philosophy:

"In March of 2000, I met a man who sat slumped on his sofa with an oxygen tube at his nose. 'Emphysema?' I asked. 'Lung cancer,' he responded. He then went on to tell me that he had received his last chemotherapy treatment and he was waiting to die. I asked him if he had considered an alternative treatment. He said that he had heard of alternative cancer treatments. I asked him, point blank, 'Do you think that your life is not worth saving?' He was very angry and said, 'That's a #### of a thing to say!' I asked him, 'Well, it's true, isn't it?' I meant no offense. I can't understand why, in the face of certain death, he would not actively pursue an alternative treatment protocol."

I know what you're thinking. That *was* a #### of a thing to say! And while I would not have approached it that way, I have complete understanding of why Bob did. It is difficult to comprehend the reasons that people will not fight for their own lives. This precious gift of breath that has been given to us seems far too valuable to let go of without a battle. I would like to think that I could not forfeit my life that easily, that I would fully engage the enemy till the end. I get the realization, however, that the true answer for many others is not that straightforward.

For probably a multitude of reasons, apparent or not, many cancer sufferers have simply given up, having perceived the battle to be lost. They may have been through the best treatments that conventional medicine has to offer with no progress, endured serious side effects, and have lived with a very poor quality of life for months or years. They are tired, very sick and, simply, have no will to continue. And add to that the fact that they are depressed, pessimistic, emotionally sterilized, and "just want it to be over." There is no more desire, no more energy, no remaining will for any additional treatments, conventional or alternative. After all, if America's "gold standard" of therapies has failed them, they cannot "visualize" that anything else could possibly work. And "where there is no vision, the people perish." Unfortunately, I've witnessed it many times. They have "seen" their death – and, suddenly, appear to be okay with it.

Many have been so heavily "treated" that they would not have survived any additional intervention, regardless of what it was. There are others, though, still upright and mobile, who might benefit from non-allopathic measures that may, at a minimum, relieve pain and give them a better quality of life for whatever time is left. Maybe, just maybe, they could still be healed. In fact, it happens everyday for many who somehow can generate the will to keep going – to keep trying – to live.

Yes, it can be said that attitude is everything. And while a good one won't necessarily heal you, a bad one will lead you rapidly in the other direction. Of this, you can be sure.

Probably one of the best statements on desire and healing comes from Ellen A. Mogensen of "Past & Now Forward Holistic Counseling":

"You are the only one who ever heals yourself. You heal for two reasons. One, you believe you deserve to heal and that belief manifests as your desire to be healed. Two, your desire to be healed manifests as action on your part to get healed. So many people delay, deny, and diffuse their healing because, at bottom, they do not want to live. The desire for healing is truly the desire for living. You will only heal if you really want to live."

Although some might consider the foregoing controversial, when you boil it down, it is unequivocally true. We usually get what we "really want" in life. This is because the things we really want are the things that we go after with all the gusto we can muster. We plan, we scheme, we cajole – we do whatever is necessary to obtain what is most important to us. And, for the most part, with this type of maximum effort, dedication, and "never quit it till I get it" attitude, the results are positive.

Thus, the "you will only heal if you really want to live" idea makes absolute sense and proves itself every day in the lives and healed bodies of those who wouldn't quit – no matter what.

You must choose the right path, however. With the best of intentions and an unequalled zest for life – you can still walk off the cliff in the darkness. Instead, seek the light with your pro life attitude; the light that reveals the truth about cancer and the treatments, therapies and protocols that work best in allowing your body to defeat this disease.

Synthetic visualization. What does that really mean? To me it has nothing to do with artificially "seeing" your cancer gone and "hoping" yourself to wellness. We get enough of synthetic things through traditional drug therapies. No, this phrase brings together, or "synthesizes", the thoughts and actions that will result in the healing of a cancerous body. And while you cannot actually "think" yourself well, you can combine a healthy and positive attitude with a tried and proven "alternative" cancer plan that will give you, without any reasonable doubt, the best chance for survival.

You'll notice that the word "alternative" is, once again, in quotation marks in the last paragraph and, largely, has been as it pertains to "Alternative Medicine" in this book. As previously stated, this term is really a misnomer in relating to the practice of non-conventional measures to bring healing to cancer patients – or any patient.

One of the best consumer advocates I know, Tim Bolen, says it best – and you need to hear it:

"'Alternative medicine' is defined as any protocol, action or therapy that isn't *drugs, radiation, or surgery oriented.*'

"Wrongfully named? Yes. So-called *alternative medicine* is actually the health choice of planet earth. It is a combination of every good health idea invented by mankind, in every country and culture on this planet. There is nothing *alternative* about it. Labeling planet earth's health choice as *alternative* is, and was, a propaganda device.

"North Americans have overwhelmingly (by their purchases) made *alternative medicine* the 'health choice of the people' – for the best of reasons: it works better than allopathic, it *removes the cause* rather than *treating the symptoms*, it is cost-effective, it makes people feel better and think clearer, and it doesn't have all those horrible effects, and side effects, of invasive surgery or prescription drugs.

"More than half of the U.S. health dollar in 1999 was spent on 'alternative medicine' and it was all out-of-pocket. Conventional medicine is being paid for, and is surviving, only because insurance and Medicare pay for it – the public won't spend an out-of-pocket nickel on it.

"Alternative medicine philosophies fit the *'American (I'll make my own decisions)'* way of thinking. Allopathic medicine philosophies fit the *'Germanic (follow my orders)'* way. *'Alternative medicine'* is for people who think for themselves – Americans.

"The door to real 'alternatives' is barely open. The future of medicine is right in front of us – it isn't in pharmaceuticals – it is in nutrition, body cleansing, prevention, oxygen therapies and energy medicine."

Gee, thanks, Tim. Exactly what is in this book. Bolen writes one of the best newsletters available – and you can get it for free. Subscribe to it at www.bolenreport.com. You'll be glad you did.

Visualize victory with your "alternative" cancer program. Understand that it is really the only way you can successfully heal. Seek out support groups and organizations. There are many that are chock full of cancer survivors who "did it their own way." Find a cancer coach, embrace (and appreciate) your advocate – even when they tell you things you "don't want to hear." Take charge of your immune-boosting therapy, exercise to get rid of the stress (if you can), embrace that "power of positive thinking" that is not an old cliché but a real life-changing process.

Yes, predict and visualize your triumph over cancer. Seeing is believing – and belief is what will get you over that last hump when it doesn't seem like anything else will.

CHAPTER TEN

"WHERE'S THE PROOF?
TESTIMONIES FROM THE LIVING;
THE EMPIRICAL REVOLUTION"

"It is amazing how quickly the tumor, for instance with colon cancer, is being eliminated. Even with an old patient of 84 years who was scheduled for an operation because of his colon threatening to become blocked, I was able to achieve the complete elimination of the tumor and the patient's restoration to health within a few days. These are not isolated cases, in fact 99% of the sick that come to see me to use the biological method of cancer therapy, are cancer patients who have had operations and radiation sessions, or who were diagnosed as being too far advanced for an operation to be of any help. Even in these cases health can be restored, usually within a few months, I would say in 90% of cases."

Dr. Johanna Budwig

"**WHERE'S** the beef?" Most of us remember the American character actress, Clara Peller, asking that question in a "Wendy's" T.V. commercial back in the early 1980's. Of course, the "beef" ended up being at "Wendy's."

Today, a similar question is being forwarded (disingenuously) by the American Medical Association (AMA), the Food and Drug Administration (FDA), and the American Cancer Society (ACS) – among others – regarding the evidence that supports the "cures" vocalized by those who have healed their cancers "naturally." They ask, with their condescending attitudes, slight smirks, and tongues firmly implanted in their cheeks, "Where's the proof?"

My response, and that of all those who represent the actual documented evidence surrounding this fiery issue, is two-fold. First, I offer, "where's *your* proof?" Where is the pile of paperwork that shows that chemotherapy, surgery, and radiation work to cure cancer? Show me the statistics – those that aren't intentionally manipulated (patients excluded that have died, cause of death listed as other than cancer, etc.) – to prove that conventional medicine is winning the war on this disease. Produce the testimonies of those who endured ten rounds of poison chemo and 30+ sessions of tissue and bone-marrow-killing radiation (sometimes over months or years) and have survived long term and their cancer hasn't returned. And, you know, while there are a few, based upon how many have been treated in this "unnatural fashion," there aren't very many.

My second response is that the empirical evidence (visible, verifiable, repeatable) for "natural cures" is overwhelming and available to all who seek it. There are thousands – probably tens of thousands – of natural healing testimonies on hundreds of websites. Communities are full of support groups filled with survivors that have used "alternative" (there's that misnomer again) methodologies – allowing their immune systems to knock out "The Big C."

That's right. You show me yours and I'll show you mine. But "you" (allopathic medicine) will have trouble producing real proof because you accept and forward *NO* proof but your own, based upon *NO* studies or clinical trials but your own. You will parade out these clinical studies which document that a few rats and mice survived the overdosing of synthetic drugs that the human body rejects. You will say that "deaths" happen during human trials and FDA-allowed drug experimentation, and that those deaths are acceptable and the price that has to be paid for better pharmaceutical agents. Like Colonel Sherman T. Potter on *M.A.S.H.,* I call "horse hockey" on all counts.

Friends, do you remember where the real proof lies? ***In the pudding!*** That's right. Not in clinical trials; not in drugs or radiation; not in the ever-expanding cancer graveyards. No, this "empirical evidence" that mainstream medicine touts as worthless, is proclaimed daily in the lives and verbal testimonies of those who are living and thriving today because they embraced the right treatments, the right therapies, and the correct protocols that the body accepts (***and requires***) to heal itself.

Are we too passive today to question why so many of our family and friends are dying of cancer? Do we not want to offend anyone? I'm sick and tired of reading the obituaries in my hometown newspaper that are filled with statements like "died after a heroic battle with cancer," and "finally passed away after a courageous, 10-year battle with cancer." Aren't you? Tell me, when do we put a stop to this? Is this a call to action? You bet it is!

The "real truth" and the "real proof" about cancer need to be "outed." Here's a myth buster concerning chemotherapy (the main cancer treatment today – the "gold standard"), revealed in an earlier chapter, and so vitally important to know and understand that it needs to be repeated:

A study, reported in the December, 2004, edition of *Clinical Oncology,* by Morgan, Ward, and Barton, on the contribution of cytotoxic chemotherapy to 5-year survival in adult malignancies, reached the following results: "The overall contribution of curative and adjuvant cytotoxic chemotherapy to 5-year survival in adults was estimated to be 2.3% in Australia and 2.1% in the USA." And, this was their conclusion: "It is clear that cytotoxic chemotherapy only makes a minor contribution to cancer survival. To justify the continued funding and availability of drugs used in cytotoxic chemotherapy, a rigorous evaluation of the cost-effectiveness and impact on quality of life is urgently required."

Now let's see, have you seen the results of that rigorous evaluation that was so "*urgently required*?" I didn't think so. And in all probability, you will not. The fact is that the proof is just *not there* to support the use of chemotherapy – or radiation – to treat cancer patients. The truth is exactly the opposite. The proof *is* there to support *ending it* once and for all. Not likely, however, given the power of the drug companies to manipulate and control their test results and the subsequent actions of the FDA. You know, I hate to have to say that. It actually "pains" me to say that. But I told you at the start that this book would be about truth – no matter what. And the real truth is that conventional medicine does not have *any* proof that their cancer protocols help cancer patients; "alternative" medicine does.

Following, you will find a small fraction of this "living proof." These testimonies are of real people telling factual stories of how they survived – many after being sent home to die by their oncologists. Please pay close attention to these. They are not fabricated, not embellished, not forced – not fairy tales. No, this is really "where the beef is, Clara."

"The long days of winter had just begun to turn, a time when life is starting to think of new beginnings. Seed catalogs show up in the mail and the crocus announce all is well. A time bomb went off in my life. I was diagnosed with inflammatory breast cancer. The pathology report read 'intralymphatic carcinoma,' explained to me as a rare and aggressive form of cancer. After my initial shock and dismay, my life flashed before my eyes. It seemed that I had two choices. I could choose life or I could choose death – they were both set before me. Then the oncologist explained that chemotherapy was the first line of defense, that my immune system would be taken down to nothing – then my body would build it back up – at which time the chemo would take it out, yet again and again. Later I would be scheduled for surgery and radiation. As hard as I tried to imagine that as 'a cure' – it seemed more like a death sentence to me.

"I decided from then on that I would choose life, and the creator of life – our Heavenly Father – would show me how to do that through the way He designed my body to heal by building up my immune system. I gave my body the tools for healing, super nutrition (100% raw) green drinks and leafy greens and vegetables that brought my body's pH to a state of alkalinity and oxygenated my cells; hot and cold showers; coffee enemas to detox; pancreatic enzyme therapy; castor oil poultice, zeolites, lots and lots of good alkaline water; infrared saunas, and mini-trampoline. The body makes between three and four million new blood cells and eleven to thirteen million body cells every second. I choose the foods and drinks that make the best blood. And Christ the Healer makes me whole. My doctor's visit and diagnosis was February 16, 2009 – over 23 months ago – I have never been back and I am well."

Gail Hartwig – Breast Cancer – Washington State

"There are no words to describe how it felt when (November '08) I was told that I had Stage 4 throat cancer with 3 months to live. 'Shocked' and 'devastated' are too mild. It was as if someone had hit me between the eyes with a brick, made me get back up, and then hit me again.

"I started with chemo (5 types over a 6-month period) and radiation (32) days. I was sick from the onset. I developed mouth sores, my hair and beard fell out, I was terribly fatigued, food had no taste, and I had lost 60 pounds in the process. But I am a fighter and I believe in God's miracles and natural healing so, in addition to chemo and radiation, I used prayer, had friends pray and SEARCHED for natural healing products.

"In May of 2009, God gave me the answer through my dear friend,

Mr. E. Johnson, who researched natural cancer cures for me. He discovered and introduced to me KANGEN 'LIVING' WATER, used in Japan for over 35 years and now available in the USA! I purchased an Enagic 'Kangen' Ionizer (the missing piece to the natural healing puzzle that I was looking for).

"Within 48 hours after drinking the Kangen Water, my mouth sores were totally gone and for the first time I could eat and drink by mouth. The doctors were in awe of my progress and thus stopped all my cancer drugs and treatments within 4 weeks because I was maintaining my health with Kangen Water.

"Since then, I have gained 20 pounds and my energy level is almost back to normal. On December 31, 2009, I received a call from my doctor to tell me that I was CANCER FREE! No more cancer in my lymph nodes, my throat, or my tongue.

"From 3 months to live…to cancer free. I believe in Kangen Water more than anything else. It has aided in my recovery and I will drink it every day for the rest of my life. It works for me. I am Living Proof."

P. P. – Throat Cancer

The following testimony is forwarded through an interview with "K.B.," a male from Missouri:

What Kind of Cancer Did You Have?
"Malignant melanoma, starting with a growth at the back and base of my neck."

How Far Had It Metastasized?
"Stage III."

What Month and Year Was It First Diagnosed?
"August, 1980 (he was 19 years old at the time)."

What Technique Did They Use to Diagnose It?
"They excised the mole and did a biopsy."

Did You Have Surgery?
"Only the excise of the mole. They wanted to do extensive surgery, such as cutting a large hole where the mole was, and to the point of removing some of my lymph nodes, but I only let them cut out the mole. They also wanted to do 3 months of chemotherapy."

Did You Take Chemotherapy or Radiation?
"No, even though I was only 19, because a friend of mine was a holistic doctor (a chiropractor) and I was aware of alternative medicine and my options – even at that time."

How Much Pressure Did the Doctors Put on You to Have Surgery, Chemotherapy, etc?
"Quite a bit, in fact, tremendous pressure. They even called my mother and got her crying."

How Long Were You Expected to Live?
"They did not give me a length."

What Was the Deciding Factor That Convinced You to Use Alternative Treatments?
"Even though I was aware of alternative medicine, I did seriously consider doing what the doctors wanted. However, I did not like their very heavy handed approach to try and force me to do the surgery and chemotherapy."

What Was the Major Alternative Treatment You Used?

"Fruit and vegetable juice diet. I studied books by Norman Walker and Paavo Airola."

What Other Alternative Treatments or Supplements Did You Take?

"My friend (the chiropractor) sold Herbalife, so I took Herbalife. He was real big on enzymes."

Please Describe Your Treatment Plan:

"First, I went on a two week fruit and vegetable juice fast (I bought a juicer the day I decided to fight the cancer on my own). During fasting, I took approximately 1 quart of carrot juice per day, often mixed with spinach, cucumber, garlic, onion, celery, etc., whatever grows. Fruit juice was usually grapes, pineapple, apple, pear, grapefruit (stayed away from oranges), approximately ½ quart in the morning; vegetable juice from noon till retiring; vegetable broth made daily in the afternoon. Also, daily lemon juice enemas (4-5 lemons per quart of water) in the morning usually after the first few days of the fast.

"Then, for one week, I ate nothing but fruits and vegetables. When not fasting, fruit juices, 1-2 pints per day; carrot/vegetable juices – approximately ½ quart per day. Then, I went on a three-week fruit and vegetable juice fast. Next, for one week, I ate nothing but fruits and vegetables, although I added nuts at this time. I did this, increasing the length of my fast, for six months. I also added more foods as I went along. The longest juice fast I went on was 37 days. Other things I did involved a lot of exercise. When I was juice fasting, I walked up to 8 miles a day. When I was eating, I jogged 40 miles every week."

Did You Ever Fear Dying?

"I always felt at peace with myself and never had a fear of dying."

Did You Eat Any Organic Foods?

"As much as I could get."

What Kind of Water Did You Drink?

"Always spring/bottled water."

What Month/Year Were You Diagnosed Cancer Free?

"At the end of six months of the raw food diet, I returned to the doctors and they declared me cancer free." (He has been in remission for over 20 years).

What Are You Doing to Stay in Remission?

"I follow the 80-20 rule. 80% of the foods I eat are raw foods. 20% are not. I also run/bike/swim at least one hour per day now and believe in a daily sauna."

How Many Medical Doctors Have You Told That You Were Cured of Cancer With Natural Foods?

"More than 10, but none were oncologists."

K.B., Missouri - Melanoma

"On January 3, 2000, I had colon cancer surgery in which 1/3 of my colon was removed. The cancer had also spread to two lymph nodes; so 14 lymph nodes were removed. I was then placed on 5-FU chemotherapy for six months. I seemed to be doing well, but six months later a blood test that was normally done once a month discovered that my CEA (carcino-embryonic antigen) level had risen to 4.6. Normal values are 0-3.0. I was then sent to U of M for a PET scan, which is a 3-dimensional scan that shows more detail than the traditional CAT scan.

"There at U of M, they discovered that the colon cancer had metasta-sized to my liver, and they also found a primary cancer on my right kidney.

I had been taking Immunocal (glutathione precursor) for a very short time. My CEA level went from 4.6 down to 3.0. I asked the doctors what this meant and I was told by the surgeon that it meant absolutely nothing. I said I did not want to have surgery until I had more tests and I wanted to find out what was going on. At U of M, it takes a long time to reschedule tests. So I don't remember exactly when I had my tests done. It was during the summer and early fall. They did say that the tumor was growing, so I did agree to have the surgery done.

"On December 23, 2001, surgery was performed on me and they removed a wedge of the left lobe of my liver and found just a watery cyst. They removed the entire right lobe of my liver, as there was a 2 X 3 cm cancerous tumor there. They removed the right kidney, which had a 2 cm primary cancer on it. They removed the adrenal gland and the gallbladder just as preventative maintenance. I was told not to take any Immunocal even after I went home from the hospital.

"In March, 2002, I had a severe toxic reaction to the 5-FU in which my blood pressure dropped to 55/40 during a blood test. I believe the Lord made sure that this did not happen to me until I was in a safe place. I was directly across the road at the Cancer Center from Gratiot Community Hospital when it suddenly dropped and I was transported to the hospital. At that time, the oncologist told me no more 5-FU – that it would kill me.

"I still have a titanium pump which was implanted at the time of surgery in my abdomen that feeds FUDR chemotherapy into my liver and I have been back on Immunocal since March (3 packets per day) during which time my weight has gone from 105 back up to the normal 120. My energy level is normal.

"I had a meeting with my liver surgeon and she said that she cannot believe how well I have done. In the beginning they had told me that with surgery and two kinds of chemotherapy I had one to two years to live. When they had actually done the surgery, they found that the cancer suddenly was not spread as far as they thought it had been. In my opinion, I honestly wonder if it had shrunk because of Immunocal. The kidney surgeon said that the cancer was not as extensive as they thought.

"Now they are saying it looks like I have been cured, but they cannot actually call it a cure until I have been cancer free for a total of five years. The colonoscopy done recently shows that there is no cancer in my colon. The CAT scan done shows that my liver has grown back to its normal size, and there is no cancer in my body. If it had not been for my friend telling me about this product at church, I believe I would not be here. I believe with all my heart and soul that the Immunocal, by raising and sustaining my glutathione levels, has built up my immune system to fight this disease."

D.M. – Metastatic Colon Cancer
From the www.immunehealthsolutions.com Website

"In June of 2008, I was diagnosed with terminal liver cancer and sent home to get my affairs in order. Because my tumor marker was in the 30,000 range, the doctor thought there may be a mistake and ordered another blood test. The new test result revealed a tumor marker over 50,000. The cancer cells were multiplying rapidly. I was given a prescription for chemotherapy but, since the insurance company would need two weeks to approve the prescription, the doctor said he did not know if I would live long enough to have it filled. It was a bleak day in my life and my wife and I left the doctor's office shattered. On the way home, we discussed how we would tell our three children this horrible news.

"The evening I was diagnosed, I was introduced to Reliv™, a nutritional product that provides optimum health to the body. I began taking Reliv™ products less than a week after I was diagnosed and almost immediately felt a difference in my body. Soon after taking a shake, I would have a short burst of energy. Within three days, a backache that I had for

20 years was gone. I was encouraged and continued to take the shakes because I knew something good was happening to my body. I began chemotherapy two weeks after my diagnosis and did not develop any of the side effects associated with the chemo. Today, my tumor marker is down to 150. I feel good and have energy even though I continue to take the chemotherapy twice every day. I also get a lot of rest each day and with the help of the optimal nutrition provided by Reliv™, my body is able to compete in the fight for my life. It has been 22 months since my battle with cancer began…the best is yet to come!"

Don Walker – Terminal Liver Cancer

(Don's continued chemotherapy is the drug called Nexavar™, in pill form, that he takes every twelve hours. It normally has horrific side effects but Don has tolerated it well so far. Obviously, his "alternative" treatment is the difference).

"My name is Suzanne Scherr Steger. I am 56 years old. I was surprised to get life changing results in recovering from cancer and chemotherapy as a result of taking the Reliv™ shakes.

"In January of 1998, I was diagnosed with aggressive breast cancer; the cancer had metastasized to the lymph nodes and was growing at a proliferation rate of 39% (17-19% is considered a fast growing cancer). I had seen my mother and her mother go through breast cancer, chemo, and radiation, and I did not want more than one experience of breast cancer. So I chose to have a double mastectomy followed by six months of experimental chemotherapy.

"Chemotherapy put me into an immediate and permanent state of menopause at age forty-four. I started shrinking due to massive bone density loss. I lost all of my hair, and I was in and out of the emergency room at the hospital so much that our family went to live with another family for 13 weeks. My blood counts had always been bad (I was chronically anemic) but during chemo, I had to have a shot of Neupogen every day to stimulate my bone marrow to produce good blood.

"In August, 1999, my doctor and I were in an open argument about my refusal to start on hormone replacement therapy. I had shrunk over an inch in the previous 12 months and had 17 prescriptions, which I could renew without his permission at the local pharmacy. He believed that the hormone replacement therapy would handle the depression, the panic attacks, and the loss of bone density. I believed that all of the prescription drugs were shortening my life, not to mention affecting the quality of life for me. I was in pain all of the time, due to residual effects of chemo-therapy, as well as the more recent slipped disks in my back. I wore a neck brace and could not stand up for more than a few minutes at a time.

"I began taking the Reliv™ shakes on October 15, 1999. For three months I took two scoops of Classic, a half a scoop of Innergize, and a full scoop of FibRestore, three times a day. For the next six weeks I added ProVantage and Soy Sentials, and took as many shakes as I could swallow. In less than five months I was off of all medications. In my first month of taking the shakes, my life-long struggle with constipation ended and I began to feel some emotional strength returning.

"After four months of taking the shakes, I had my regularly-scheduled oncology visit. My blood counts were perfect and my oncologist encour-aged me to keep doing whatever it was that I was doing. He said that he could not have told from my blood work that I had ever been sick. At six months, my chronically low blood pressure and tunnel vision went away. At twelve months, a bone density scan proved that my 47-year-old bones had the density of a 30-year-old woman."

Suzanne Steger – Breast Cancer

"My name is Greg Hainer. I live in Dodge City, Kansas, where I'm employed as a plumber and operate a small family farm.

"In June of 2003, I was diagnosed with colo-rectal cancer. During the surgery to remove that tumor, it was discovered that the cancer had spread and was at stage four; they found several tumors on my liver and cancer in my lymphatic system.

"My first visit with the oncologist was unquestionably the most difficult day of my life. The doctor told me that the only thing he could do at that point was to treat me with chemotherapy in hopes of slowing the cancer down, but he made it very clear to me that it was only a matter of time before the side effects of those drugs would force them to stop the treatments and that there would be nothing more they could do for me. With a wife and two young daughters at home, I think the hardest thing to accept was that I would not be there for my family and live long enough to watch my girls grow up. Just a few days later, I was told about the Reliv™ nutrition and, out of desperation, I began taking the products, although my doctor strongly advised against it.

"Three months after starting chemotherapy and taking my first Reliv™ shake, CT scans were done to see if there were any changes in the tumors on my liver. Amazingly, they could not find any cancer in my body. My doctor could not believe this had happened and even today, almost seven years later, he still cannot explain why the cancer was gone so quickly and why it has never returned.

"There is no doubt in my mind that through answered prayer and superior nutritional products, my body was able to not only overcome the cancer, but continues to keep it from returning.

"The greatest gift of all came just a few years later when I was able to watch our oldest daughter walk across the stage and receive her high school diploma. I was there when our youngest daughter graduated from the 8th grade and entered high school. And now I have the opportunity to share this incredible sense of hope with so many people. What a gift I have been given."

Greg Hainer – Metastatic Colon Cancer

"My name is Dena Guidice and I want to share with you how Transfer Factor™ has saved my life. In November of 1998, I was diagnosed with lung cancer. At that time, my team of doctors recommended that the best course of treatment for my cancer would be to perform radiation and chemotherapy simultaneously. I got started with both treatments immediately and was given the highest dosages of treatment possible. Over the next 90 days, I suffered from all of the normal side effects including weakness, vomiting, hair loss and severe weight loss. My radiation and chemo treatments ended late February, 1999.

"On March 25th, 1999, I went in for surgery (as planned), and the doctors removed a tumor from my right lung along with the top 1/3 of my lung and three sections of my ribs. The surgery went very well, and the doctors believed that they had successfully removed all of the cancer from my body. After my surgery, I went through an additional 12 weeks of chemotherapy from May to July, 1999, as a "safety measure." It was during this time that my body became so weak that all I could do was sleep and lie in bed all day. I lost all of my hair at this point and my fingernails and teeth became so brittle that I started to lose them as well. I lost my appetite completely and got to the point where I weighed only 88 pounds.

"Even as sick as I was in the summer, I was still hopeful that by fall I would get stronger after the chemotherapy was out of my system. My hope was short lived, however. In August, I found a lump under my left arm. After another surgery to remove that tumor, the tests confirmed that I had malignant lymphatic cancer (cancer of the lymph nodes) and that the cancer was all over my whole body. At that point in time, my team of doctors told me there was nothing they could do for me. I had Stage 4 (final stage) cancer and I had a maximum of 4 to 6 months to live. They told me to do everything I've always wanted to do in life within the next 45-60 days because, after that, I would be much too weak and too sick to do anything whatsoever. By this time, I was convinced that I was going to die – especially since the doctors had never seen a person live beyond 8 months – in my condition with my kind of cancer.

"At this point, I shared the devastating news with my kids, and we all took a trip to Hawaii. In my own mind, I knew that this would be my 'farewell trip.' I had given up every ounce of hope, and I had mentally prepared myself to die. It was at this time (1st week in October) that my son finally convinced me to start taking Transfer Factor™. In my mind, I was 100% convinced that it wouldn't do anything for me but, nonetheless, I started taking six Transfer Factor Plus™ and six regular Transfer Factor™ capsules every day. Within 30 days, I started to feel a little stronger and regained my appetite, but I still believed in my mind that my life was soon to be over. I kept taking the product. By January, 2000, about 90 days after starting on Transfer Factor™, I found myself even stronger and had gained back 7 pounds.

"I continued taking Transfer Factor™ every day. It's now been 7 months since I started taking Transfer Factor™ (May, 2000). I've now gained a total of 26 pounds and I feel healthier than I've felt in over 2 years. I just went to see my doctor 2 weeks ago and he said that, 'I'm a living Miracle' and that I have no signs of cancer. Transfer Factor™ has not only saved my life, it has given me hope for tomorrow and the years ahead."

Dena Guidice – Metastatic Lung Cancer

"When I was only 27, I received the terrifying news that I had Hodgkin's Disease. I was devastated. The tumor in my chest cavity was so large that it completely filled my entire rib cage. I began on chemotherapy. At that time, my immune system was down to 2000 points. I had a friend who I knew could help me with nutrition. Mike recommended several supplements to strengthen my immune system. Then, Mike introduced me to transfer factors and I began to take 12 a day.

"Much to my doctor's surprise, my immune system began to go up. In fact, it went all the way BACK up to 7200. The doctors said that they had never, ever seen anyone's immune system go UP during chemotherapy. Well, then the chemotherapy began to fry, literally fry my lungs, so they had to discontinue it. Amazingly, while off of the chemo, and on the transfer factors, my tumor continued to shrink. Again, the doctors were shocked, but I went ahead and took radiation with my immune system staying up!! Now I am taking transfer factors and enhanced transfer factors. My tumor is completely GONE, and I am 30 years old. I have been free of cancer for over 10 months. This is not just a necessary product for everyone; it is something I will never be without."

Ann L. – Hodgkin's Lymphoma

"I will shortly be celebrating the second anniversary of my becoming a RAW VEGETARIAN. It was about two years ago, at the height of my suffering from deadly cancer, that I was introduced to the raw-food diet, which completely changed my life. In fact, it saved my life. Today, after nineteen months of eating raw vegetable food, I am a completely different person. I have not used any medicine since about a year before becoming a Raw Vegetarian and I feel very healthy. My right arm, which had been completely numb since the breast operation, has become normal. For the first time in more than three years, I felt my arm itching. I really cried for joy. I will never forget that moment."

Maryam Neshan Barjan (Maria), Teheran, Iran
From the www.healingcancernaturally.com Website

"In 1996, my husband's routine physical checkup at the VA hospital revealed a tumor in one of his lungs. The doctors wanted to perform a biopsy immediately to find out if the growth was malignant and they were already talking about radiation and chemo "therapy." From past experience and knowledge, I knew that this was not the answer. These so-called 'therapies' provide no hope for real cure. Biopsies are very traumatic to the body and chemo/radiation are well known to destroy the immune system.

"Instead, I immediately began to treat my husband (Chuck) with Homeopathy, raw vegetable juice, flaxseed oil, herbal formula in tincture/extract form such as the Essiac formula, the Hoxsey formula, and Cat's Claw extract.

"Since 1996, doctors have continued to monitor Chuck's tumor with their CAT scan and PET scan. The tests revealed that a small mass still remains in his lung, but the doctors aren't concerned about it because the tumor has completely stopped growing and Chuck experiences none of the usual symptoms associated with lung cancer. To this day he remains healthy and well."

Shirley Lipschutz-Robinson, © 2002
www.shirleys-wellness-café.com (great site)

"Two days after Christmas in 2008, a chest x-ray revealed that I had a large tumor (9 cm.) the size of my fist…at which time I began to dramatically increase my Reliv shakes. On January 6th, 2009, a surgical biopsy was done and we learned that I had lymphoma, which was later classified and staged. Since an initial PET scan revealed that there was evidence of it on both sides of my diaphragm, the label they gave me was "Non-Hodgkin's (Large B Cell) Lymphoma, Stage 3"…which was not good news.

"The treatment program that was recommended for me is called R-CHOP, and it is considered strong chemotherapy. R-CHOP is a combination of Rituxin along with Cytoxan, Adriamycin, Vincristine, and Prednisone, a really nasty combination of drugs. My first round of chemo was on January 22nd, and I took Reliv the entire time that I was on chemotherapy, even *during* my infusions. I mention that because it would have been very difficult for me to do that by myself; my wife would mix my shakes and hand me one about every two hours while I was receiving my treatments. We did this because we felt that I needed to get just as much good nutrition into my body as I could while I was receiving chemotherapy through my infusions. Well, that paid off, because less than three months later, on April 17, 2009, my oncologist told me that a second PET scan revealed no cancerous activity whatsoever! What had been Stage 3 Lymphoma was no longer Stage 2, or even Stage 1. My oncologist declared me to be in full remission, and I will be scanned periodically for the next 5 years just as a precaution.

"There is no doubt in my mind that strong chemotherapy literally dissolved the malignant tumors in my body, but the problem with chemotherapy is that it destroys more than just cancer cells, it also kills things you need, things like healthy cells. Reliv helped my body create healthy cells and it allowed me to withstand the ravages of strong chemotherapy. The entire time that I was on chemotherapy, my blood work was perfect – red cell count, white cell count, platelet count, you name it. I never experienced any fatigue, no nausea, no constipation, no neuropathy, no mouth sores and, really, no pain of any kind. The whole litany of side-effects that they told me were coming my way never, ever materialized. I never missed a day of work, which was truly a blessing and, really, my only side-effect throughout my ordeal was hair loss and, of course, it has all grown back. Most people that have taken strong chemotherapy will tell you that their experience was not at all like mine.

"I think what amazed my oncologist the most is that *I never missed a day of work* and, when he discharged me in May, 2009, my oncologist described my recovery as both 'dramatic and remarkable.' I credit God's grace, lots of answered prayers, and the power of patented nutrition. I refer to it as the **ultimate** hat trick!

"The Reliv products do **not** cure cancer, I want to be very clear about that. But when you put the best possible nutrition into the human body – faithfully and consistently – the human body can do amazing things. It can heal – just as God designed it to do."

Cliff Bachman, Engineer, St. Louis, Missouri

"My father was about 45 years old when he was diagnosed with eczema by his physician. He was treated with a skin cream and told to just keep the area dry. However, after several months the affected area increased in size and the doctor recommended he use a heat light to help treat the condition.

"After several years, the symptoms slowly became worse with open areas that had drainage. The location involved was a large region around his waist. He changed doctors several times trying to find someone that could heal his skin condition.

"My mother was a practicing health nutritionist, self-educated. She was always encouraging us to eat plenty of fruits and vegetables. I encouraged my father to get another opinion after showing me the diseased area that now had a strong odor – indicating to me that it was probably cancer. The doctor then admitted my father immediately to a hospital in Chicago. The blood work showed that my father had advanced cancer and was treated with radiation.

"My mother would brew herb teas and bring them to him at the hospital. The herbs she used were Red Clover, Chaparral, Devil's Claw and Burdock Root. The results amazed the doctors and especially the head of dermatology. His doctor would ask him each day what he was doing. My father was uncomfortable telling him that his wife came each morning with a thermos full of tea. The doctor came in a few days later and told my father that it was not what they were doing – but something else that was healing him. His skin became as a 'newborn's skin' that 'they could not credit to the results of radiation.' The head of the department told my father that it was what he (my father) was doing that healed his cancer. My father also took large doses of vitamin C and vitamin E with selenium daily.

"Before my father was discharged from the hospital about a week later, blood work showed that he did not have one cancer cell in his blood. He continued to live a healthy and active life and never had a recurrence of cancer."

Holly Swardstrom, R.N., Washington

"I had just been diagnosed and told that I had the precursor of prostate cancer. My PSA was at 13.5 and rising. My doctor wanted to be aggressive with this and I had already watched my father go through surgery, chemo, and radiation with this same disease. It was not pretty to watch as my dad had been healthy his entire life – he never got sick – and had even boxed for the Navy and had many trophies to show for it. The prostate cancer 'broke' my dad; he went from being a strong healthy man to catching everything that came by and his quality of life changed dramatically. I did not want that so, yes, I gave the presenter at the Kangen Water presentation I was attending my undivided attention. I sat up in my chair, followed what was being said and shown – and started drinking the water. The folks working the room kept my glass full. I noticed that night that, with all the water I had consumed, I wasn't running to the bathroom to get rid of any – that was interesting to me.

"The next day I started getting Kangen Water from the lady who is now my mentor. I started that the last week of February, 2009. At that time I was taking medication for diabetes, acid reflux, gastritis, high blood pressure, asthma, allergies (including one to gluten), post-traumatic stress disorder (PTSD), sinusitis, migraines – a total of 19 prescription drugs including insulin. I was taking drugs for the ailments and drugs for the side-effects. I also wore dark glasses for the inside and darker glasses for the outside due to a light sensitivity I developed during one of my Army assignments. I suffered with that sensitivity from January, 1974, until 12 days after I began drinking Kangen Water.

"The first change I noticed was my light sensitivity disappeared and I didn't get migraines any more. On July 27, 2009, my primary care doctor removed me from 14 of the prescriptions – including insulin. He was surprised at my numbers and wanted to know what I did. I told him the only thing I changed was the type and amount of water I drank. He was skeptical so I gave him information about Kangen Water and all he said to me was, 'Keep doing whatever you are doing.' Next, I went to my urologist/oncologist and requested another screening be done. He didn't want to do it but I asked him to humor me. He did the test and could not believe the results. One more prescription gone and today I still have my prostate and my PSA readings are hanging around 3 and 4. YES!!! The only medications I stayed on were the four for my PTSD.

"As I write this, my psychiatrist has removed me from an anxiety drug – I'm down to three now for my PTSD. I feel great and can't wait to relieve my body of the psychotropic drugs I'm still taking. *The only thing I have changed during all this time is that I drink lots of Kangen Water*. It has really changed my quality of life.

"Unfortunately, my dad's PSA continues to rise – now at 27 – and he's refusing any treatment and, since he has a very high pain threshold – we can't tell when he is in pain. Hospice is working with him."

Jay – Bellingham, Washington

"In 2001, I was diagnosed with Hodgkin's Lymphoma while expecting my third child. I went through treatments (chemo and radiation) and I thank God that my baby was born healthy – five weeks prematurely. I was in excruciating pain 24 hours a day from the side effects of the treatments which caused many additional health problems, such as difficulty breathing because of severe damage caused to my lungs, hot flashes, heart palpitations, headaches, chest pains, and pain in my muscles, legs, and feet. They killed my thyroid with radiation treatments, so I was put on Synthroid medication. I was finally able to stop taking this drug and have now, thankfully, been off of it for six years. In the beginning, the doctors told me not to take Reliv because its soy ingredients would react to the Synthroid – but now they tell me not to go off of it because it's helped stimulate my thyroid to make it work again.

"In January, 2003, I had a CT scan and they found spots on my lungs again. My husband and I prayed for a miracle. That's when I was introduced to Reliv. I was desperate for anything by this point and I'd already tried many vitamins from health food stores, many different supplements, and was still weak with no improvements to show from these products. Reliv became the answer to our prayers.

"In March of 2003, I started taking the basic nutritional supplements offered by Reliv and noticed an improvement almost immediately. I had more energy and stamina right away. In two weeks I was pain free and slept the whole night through – which was a first in a long time. I had undergone one carpal tunnel operation because of side effects from my previous treatments and was scheduled for the second one but – thankfully – didn't end up needing it. Things finally started looking up and within three months the cancer was in remission.

"I was diagnosed with breast cancer in April of 2007, when I became so busy with moving and family that I slacked off on my nutritional shakes.

The doctors had originally told me that the Hodgkin's Lymphoma treatments would eventually be followed by breast cancer and that it would be stage four within four weeks of diagnosis. I immediately started taking more and more Reliv shakes and discovered at the four-week check-up that the cancer had shrunk in half. Six weeks later they gave me the good news that it had shrunk in half again and the lesions around the tumor were 75%-80% gone or invisible. The doctor was shocked but still kept insisting on surgical methods. Instead, I did check-ups every two months until it had all shrunk away."

Deborah Weaver – Grottoes, Virginia

"In July of 2009, I felt like I was falling apart. At the age of thirty-one, I was suffering from high blood pressure, hypothyroid disorder, anemia, fatigue, migraines, and insomnia. Everyday I struggled to take care of my busy family. With five children, I barely had time to blink. Taking a 'sick day' was not an option. Then, in late July, my doctor diagnosed me with cervical cancer and I just wanted to scream with frustration. I knew I needed to get serious about my nutrition. I began taking the Reliv nutritional products that August.

"After two weeks, I noticed I was no longer having migraines. My energy improved and I was sleeping better than I had slept in years. My husband was enjoying better sleep as well and our children were begging for their shakes every morning. A few weeks later, my blood work showed I was no longer anemic. I felt great!

"I was feeling great and my family was thrilled. We started to dream again. We began envisioning a future doing the things we had always wanted to do. Then, from out of left field, a curve ball was thrown my direction. I began having seizures, blinding pain behind my eyes, and vision problems. An MRI revealed a brain tumor that had previously gone unnoticed.

"I continued taking my Reliv shakes everyday. In January, 2010, I was told the cervical cancer was no longer an issue. In fact, my doctor could find no trace of the cancer during a physical exam or in my blood work. I was elated! However, I was still struggling with the debilitating effects of the brain tumor.

"Then, in February, we chose to have surgery to remove the tumor in my brain. During pre-surgical scans, the doctors found something very unexpected. The tumor had dissolved itself! All they could find was a pocket of fluid where the tumor had been with some garbage cells. Amazing! We chose to have surgery, placing a shunt to drain the fluid. I was told it would take six months to recover from the swelling on my brain. Just three months later, I was up, chasing after my five kids again and no longer needed a nap in the afternoon. My doctors were amazed and my family was ecstatic!

"Today, I am happy to say, I have my life back and a quality of life I thought was lost. My whole family takes the Reliv nutritional products and would not stop if someone paid us."

Shiloh W., Troy, Missouri

With the permission of my good friend, Jessica Biscardi, I submit her testimony as told through the television special series, *The Incurables*, by Veria T.V:

The daughter of actress, singer, and dancer, Marquita Rivera, and fashion photographer, Eugene Biscardi, Jessica Biscardi is a former model and Ms. New York. She is an actress who has been featured in television episodes of *Fantasy Island, Judging Amy, The X-Files,* among others – and has also appeared in several movies including *Geronimo: An American Legend.*

Jessica was diagnosed with four invasive carcinomas and given only one to three months to live unless she underwent intense chemotherapy and radiation treatments. Her breast cancer had metastasized to her lymph system, her pancreas, and lungs. Doctors also wanted her to submit to a double mastectomy. She refused. She did have a biopsy and four lymph nodes removed – then decided to deal with her cancer nutritionally after a bout with the drugs Tamoxifen and Arimidex produced seven mini-strokes.

Under the supervision of medical doctor and oncologist, James Forsythe, naturopathic doctor, Bernardo Majalca, biochemist, Vincent Gammill, and internist and medical doctor, David Schiff, Jessica began her journey of natural healing. With assistance from her daughter and husband, Jessica undertook a regimen of natural foods and juices and eliminated sugars, dairy, and red meat from her diet. Additionally, she started I.V. treatments with the natural supplement Poly-MVA through Dr. Forsythe, then continued this protocol through oral doses eight times a day upon returning home.

After about six months, Jessica's pH had risen to about 7.3 and MRI and CT scans showed "no neoplastic disease present." She later learned that she had hypothyroidism and discovered that the chemotherapy that her doctors had recommended she commence immediately – may well have killed her.

Jessica Biscardi is alive and well today because she resisted the pressure to do the universally accepted and doctor-directed, convenient thing – and did the "right thing" instead.

Following are profiles of cancer patients who were success-fully treated at Camelot Cancer Care in Tulsa, Oklahoma:

Patient #1 – Non-Hodgkin's Lymphoma, B cell, Burkitt's form (in his own words – initials L.L.)

"I was the first patient treated by Camelot Cancer Care for Non-Hodgkin's Lymphoma. They have treated many others since that time. The report of my gallium scan of August 20, 1999, metastatic disease progression (abnormal uptake in adenopathy) was by then evident in my groin, plus also the left clavicle and three regions of my spine (actual first diagnosis was 1997).

"My oncologist, Dr. Miller, had predicted my likely death from this disease within an estimated 3 months, unless I submitted to localized radiation treatment, plus chemotherapy. My research determined that radiation would result in impotence and incontinence, so I refused. When I asked Dr. Miller for contact with Non-Hodgkin's Lymphoma patients who had undergone the chemo and radiation treatment he was proposing, he admitted that none in my age bracket had survived the methotrexate and cytosine arabinocide. There was something wrong with this picture – I would die if I didn't, yet everyone in my age bracket was killed by it.

"I elected to pursue the DMSO option. My IV treatments took a couple of hours each and I had them three times weekly (M-W-F) for three weeks, for a total of nine treatments. Two weeks after my final treatment, I reported for a PET scan, in early August of 2000, to see if we had made any headway. To my great surprise, that report showed no evidence of any metastatic disease process anywhere within my body. That was almost ten years ago, and I have remained in good health with no symptoms of NH Lymphoma recurrence.

"I was talking to a pathologist at a lab in Hollywood, Florida, a few days ago and he related to me how his lab had done testing for cancer markers on a Non-Hodgkin's Lymphoma patient being treated at Vanderbilt University, a big teaching hospital in Nashville, Tennessee. The treating oncologist called him, and when he asked what chemo the Non-Hodgkin's Lymphoma patient was receiving, the oncologist replied 'methotrexate.' The pathologist asked the oncologist if he was aware that metho-trexate causes brain lesions and bleeding.

"He replied 'yes, but it's the standard of care for Non-Hodgkin's Lymphoma.' The pathologist then asked if he could administer DMSO, as it would reduce brain swelling, heal the lesions caused by the methotrexate, and is known to cure malignancy also. The oncologist replied his hospital IRB (Institutional Review Board) would not meet for another two months, and would be unlikely to approve such an alternative, 'off-the-wall' treatment in lieu of the standard. You guessed it, the patient was just allowed to die. He was an extremely wealthy and powerful man, too. It made no difference. Anyway, I just found out a few weeks ago that metho-trexate causes lesions and bleeding within the brain, and often the Non-Hodgkin's Lymphoma patient dies from this treatment, not his cancer.

"I write to you because, as a survivor of this terrible disease, I want to encourage others to take the path I did and not give in to the poisonous chemo and radiation which conventional doctors use to treat cancer. I asked Camelot Cancer Care to notify me of any potential patient who has Non-Hodgkin's Lymphoma or any other form of this terrible disease so that I can share my experience and perhaps keep them from the very uncomfortable, worthless treatment practiced by conventional doctors. The side effects of losing the hair, nausea, and other discomfort does not happen with the DMSO treatment. It is very comfortable with no side effects or discomfort of any kind. I can't understand why the doctors in every country are not using this miracle treatment. But, of course, it is not patentable so there is no profit for the large drug companies, I am sure.

"During this crusade of mine, I have talked to many, many other cancer patients with all kinds of cancer, and the treatment at Camelot has been successful in curing many, if not most, of them. This is especially true if they have not had their immune systems completely destroyed by the chemo and radiation. It has now been over thirteen years since my original cancer diagnosis, and I have outlived one of the doctors who made dire predictions of my death if I did not undergo chemo and radiation. Looking back on it now, refusing was one of the smartest things I ever did. I will be 79 next month. I am well past the 5-year survival date and am still in good health. My letter to a Veteran's Administration oncologist, who wanted to know the details of how I survived a late stage, aggressive malignancy that they consider terminal, is posted on Camelot's web site. I was their first patient and so am the longest one to survive cancer free. Mainstream oncology calls my case a 'lucky fluke,' but luck had nothing to do with it – it was the DMSO."

L.L's testimony is the longest in this series and is a clear example of the efficacy of DMSO and the failure of conventional medicine and drug therapies.

Patient #2– Glioblastoma (brain tumor, grim prognosis, generally considered terminal)

Jim Prescott (name changed) is a 58-year-old male, retired federal agent, living in Tennessee. He had no pertinent medical history prior to his diagnosis. Jim had complained only of blurred vision and a feeling of pressure behind his eyes, which led to his doctor ordering an MRI scan. It revealed a left posterior parietal brain lesion. He had surgery the next day; craniotomy to debulk, with subtotal resection (meaning they could not get it all). Biopsy confirmed it was a high grade, aggressive malignancy. Chemo and radiation were offered, but Jim declined and started on intravenous DMSO/Laetrile treatment at Camelot when he was 3 ½ weeks post-op. He received three 20-day rounds of IV DMSO based formula, a total of 60 consecutive days. His post treatment PET scan indicated his malignancy was resolved; there was no evidence of recurrent or residual tumor activity. His video testimonial is posted on Camelot's website at www.camelotcancercare. com.

Patient #3 – Colon Cancer

"My name is Ursula Simmons (name changed) and I was diagnosed with adenocarcinoma of the ascending colon in July of 2005. I went to CTCA (Cancer Treatment Centers of America – in Tulsa, OK) with the intent of having surgery, and was not informed that I was in Stage 3 (lymph node positive, with 85% chance of recurrence) until I awoke from surgery. I was told the next step was chemo.

"But, having seen the results of chemo with family and friends, I knew it was not something I wanted to go through. At the time I went to CTCA, I was under the impression that they offered alternative medicine. I was not aware that it was actually 'integrative' medicine, meaning the use of surgery, chemo, radiation, as well as nutrition, acupuncture, etc. The point being – that chemo and radiation played a big part in their medical protocol. I was to learn that natural, alternative treatments like DMSO were not offered nor sanctioned by CTCA. I only found out about DMSO through other cancer patients who were receiving it.

"I chose DMSO as my only course of treatment following my surgery. I've had a total of 11 treatments and have never taken any drugs of any kind for the cancer. On November 28, 2005, I chose to have a PET scan done to confirm what I already knew by then. No sign of cancer was the result.

"I know DMSO is something we are not taught as a method to deal with cancer. But when I looked at all the people I knew that did use the conventional method we are taught to use, I felt I didn't have a choice but to give my body a better chance to fight on its own.

"I don't regret my choice. Maureen and the Camelot staff are truly interested in helping people. I trust them and I would tell anyone, DMSO should be the first choice, not the last, because before you undergo standard chemo and radiation, your body still has somewhat of an immune system."

Ursula is now over 5 years "cancer free."

Patient #4 – Sarcoma in the left thigh region

Jerry North (name changed) is a 38-year-old male Network Operating Engineer from Texas, married father of four. His original tumor was surgically removed in October of 2008. The surgical pathology report confirmed sarcoma, and it recurred, as is usually the case with this notoriously aggressive form of malignancy. He started treatment at Camelot in November of 2009. Jerry describes his experience as follows: "My hair never fell out, I have never vomited or experienced any pain from my treatment with DMSO. The only side effect – I smelt like a mixture of garlic/corn. Currently, I still feel wonderful. I received the initial 21-day treatment of DMSO with other ingredients including

Vitamin D3, Laetrile, etc. I also was treated with Coley's Toxins, UVBI (ultraviolet blood irradiation), hyperthermia, sauna with ozone, artemesinin, and radio frequencies. I followed up with more take home treatments through my PICC line access. The tumor is still there, but I believe it will eventually be dissolved by my body if I continue alternative treatments, and as long as I address the causes of cancer and not simply the symptoms. I continue life normally. I am the Cub master in Boy Scouts. I ride bikes, camp, garden, run, jump…I am a rarity out in public as I never see anyone else with PICC lines like mine, out and about, shopping, getting groceries, etc. I am alive and well."

Patient #5 – Appendiceal/Ovarian Carcinoma

Lorraine Neal (name changed) is a 39-year old retail store manager with Stage IV, recurrent appendiceal/ovarian carcinoma, biopsy confirmed. She was first diagnosed in 2002 when she underwent surgery for acute appendicitis. Surgery and pathology reports revealed adenocarcinoma of the appendix with perforation of the small intestine, and progression to the uterus, ovaries, peritoneum and omentum.

The patient underwent radical hysterectomy and colostomy in October of 2007, contracted VRE (Vancomycin-Resistant Enterococcus) in the ICU, and her urine was found to have a heavy concentration of candida albicans, which is a typical finding in most cancer patients. Lorraine had extensive standard chemotherapy post-op, but by December of 2009, scans revealed both lung and liver nodules (the latter were successfully resected). She began DMSO/B17 based intravenous treatment at Camelot on January 18th of 2010. She also received not only Coley's Toxins and UVBI (Ultraviolet Blood Irradiation – aka photoluminescence) but, at her brother's insistence, she was treated with every weapon in Camelot's alternative arsenal.

Her colostomy has now been taken down (reversed, with reconnection). Her recent PET scan was negative, much to the joy and relief of Lorraine and her family. Most significant was the radiologist's note on her report that he found "no evidence of former cancer activity in the liver." It should be noted that Dimethylsulfoxide (DMSO), when administered intravenously, saturates all soft tissues throughout the body, including, of course, lungs and liver. It also crosses the blood/brain barrier. It leaves nowhere for cancer cells to hide.

Patient #6 – Pediatric Glioblastoma

Little 3-year old Kenny McKnight's parents brought him to Camelot from their home in rural Kansas. He had been diagnosed with glioblastoma. The tumor had been surgically debulked but he had not had chemotherapy nor radiation as yet. Having seen the other children who had undergone the burning and poisoning, only to have their cancers return, his parents were not open to it.

Kenny was back in a stroller and diapers (at age 3), the brain tumor having taken its toll. He could no longer run and play with his brother, nor even toilet himself. Fortunately, he had a porta-cath recently installed by the surgeons who had debulked (removed most of) his brain tumor mass. This intravenous access had been placed by the mainstream hospital in expectation that Kenny's parents would comply with the pediatrician's demand that he submit to chemotherapy soon after the surgery.

But his parents failed to appear at the hospital at the appointed time with little Kenny, even though the doctor had ordered his chemo to start on that morning. Instead, they had traveled to Camelot Cancer Clinic in Tulsa, where treatment had begun with intravenous DMSO-based formula. Kenny tolerated it well and soon began to respond. After a few days, his mother returned to work in Kansas while his father stayed behind with him in Tulsa.

Several days into Kenny's treatment, his mother called his father in a panic, saying Kenny's pediatrician had notified child welfare authorities of the parent's refusal to bring him in for chemo-therapy. The social workers were accompanied by agents from the Kansas State Bureau of Investigation and they had a warrant for custody of the child.

Camelot's administrator, Maureen Long, got the name of the pediatrician and her fax number and had the parents sign-off on a letter formally terminating her (pediatrician) from their child's care. It was then faxed to the doctor being fired with a copy to the mother at the home address who, subsequently, handed it to the waiting officers of the Court. They all looked it over, made calls, and were advised that the parents had a right to fire the pediatrician from the case and choose alternative treatment for their child. The state officials were without authority to step in since, clearly, there was no neglect – the child WAS receiving treatment out of state.

Kenny's treatment at Camelot continued and his little body responded. After two 20-day rounds of DMSO-based intrave-nous care (about six weeks), Kenny abandoned his stroller and began walking again and going to the bathroom by himself. He not only recovered his toilet training and his legs, he could talk again. The post-treatment PET scan showed that his residual brain tumor (the portion that the surgeons could not reach) HAD RESOLVED. Two years have now passed. Kenny is a normal, healthy little boy, ready to start kindergarten in the fall.

The following three testimonies are from individuals who have been through treatment at the Hope4Cancer Institute in Mexico. Their names have been changed but their stories remain valid and life-changing:

"I have always been a believer in Alternative Medicine and, after meeting with doctors in this country, my gut feeling was that I definitely needed alternative care. I know it was divine guidance that led me to Dr. Tony. We toured seven different clinics and it led me to choose the Hope4Cancer Clinic and Dr. Antonio Jimenez. His approach was confident, optimistic, loving, and caring.

"Dr. Tony not only saved my life, but he saved the quality of my life. It has been nine months, I am cancer free and do not have a colostomy bag! He worked hard to give me back my whole, complete life, and I am now able to do all the things I did before having cancer. I didn't know how sick I was until I started feeling better. My fast recovery is the result of the excellent care I received from all the doctors, nurses and staff who lovingly took part in my healing."

Andrea McCall – Colon Cancer

"I was diagnosed with an ovarian cancer tumor the size of a melon and you were the first call that I made. You told me to have the tumor removed and to send the pathology and surgical reports to you as soon as possible. As soon as I received the reports, they were in your hands. My oncologist here in the States assumed that I would be doing chemo but I knew in the fiber of my being that chemo would not be the right choice for me. So off we went to visit the clinic in Mexico.

"After discussing my case with you, we developed a treatment program. I was to do the SPDT (Sono-Photo Dynamic Therapy) program along with the anti-cancer vaccine injections, Poly-MVA, Immunocare, and the Total Oral Health Program. I was trained over the course of a day and a half on how to do the program at home. Once we were set up with the full spectrum lighting, my treatments began. I must say that the SPDT program is very relaxing as well as effective. Over the next few weeks, we watched my CA 125 plummet. All of my doctors were monitoring my lab results through CA 125 reports and CT scans and, with each result, the news was getting better and better. There was no cancer to be found. I couldn't be happier!"

Teri Horner – Ovarian Cancer

"Shortly after the second surgery, a new tumor appeared and the doctors in South Africa offered little hope even if chemotherapy, radiation and a third surgery were to be performed. The Hope4Cancer medical team took on this very tough challenge and provided me with a non-toxic treatment approach. I am now 4 years post-treatment and living a normal life, enjoying the company of my elder sister, younger brother, and loving parents."

Vincent Cook – Brain Tumor

It is probable that one of the most compelling testimonies for alternative treatments comes to us from across the "pond." At the following link you can read the saga of little **Bobby Wright** who was diagnosed at the age of three with a rare type of bone cancer. This inspiring story is told by Bobby's father, Kevin Wright, through a speech delivered recently at the 35th Annual Cancer Control Society Convention. Following is an excerpt from his address:

"I could not believe that Bobby might have cancer, but it was something that I had to get my head around. Denial would help no one.

"The biopsies and CT were carried out and, the next day, we were called to an office and, upon entering, Jackie immediately started crying. There was a new doctor on the team in the room. Jackie knew that he was an oncologist, as she had worked in that hospital as a nurse before we started our family.

"The doctor said that Bobby had stage 4 neuroblastoma, with metastases to bones and marrow. His primary tumor site was his left adrenal. The tumor was bi-lobed and seven centimeters by eight centimeters, but it had spread into every bone marrow cavity – into his skull bone – and he had two further tumors on his left femur.

"I was so very, very angry. The four-week misdiagnosis was unforgivable, but I now know that many parents take their kids to doctors dozens of times over a twelve or even eighteen month period before a neuroblastoma diagnosis is made – because its such a rare cancer. I asked, 'What's the survival rate for this neuroblastoma?' I was told under 20% survived one year and 3% survived for five.

"'What caused this?' I asked. 'No one knows,' was the reply. 'There's no money going into researching causes.' 'What can I do to improve his chances?' 'Nothing,' was the reply. 'What about diet?' They said there's no evidence that diet makes any difference at all. We should let Bobby eat whatever he wants to reduce the inevitable weight loss.

"Now, I'm not stupid, yet these people were obviously wrong. So I said, 'O.K. then. So we take Child A. We give him a Burger King for breakfast, a KFC for lunch, McDonald's for dinner, plenty of Pringles, lots of Diet Coke. And then we take Child B, and feed him a diet based around home-cooked food. Are you telling me that they will do the same?' The answer was the same again. 'There's no evidence to show that there would be any difference in outcome.'

"Now I was already steamingly, ragingly furious, and to be told such complete and utter rubbish just added to my fury. I just refused to believe that, with the technology available in the 21st Century, we couldn't at least have an educated guess on causes. As far as diet is concerned, the U.K. health authorities had been spending millions of pounds on education to tell us that we should eat at least five portions of fruit and vegetables a day.

"I ended the meeting right there, right then, as to argue with these people was obviously pointless."

To get the full story of little Bobby Wright – and what eventually became of him – visit the link below.

www.embracinghealth.com.au/news/bobbyscancer.pdf

I steadfastly believe that, should all similar testimonies (as aforementioned) be catalogued into reference books, a small town library would not hold them. We began this segment by referring to "empirical" evidence. It is defined *(Wikipedia)* as "evidence or research that derives its data by means of direct observation, experiment, or experience. Its results are based on actual evidence as opposed to theory or conjecture." In other words, it bases its explanations on what can be directly observed in a replicable or repeatable manner.

There are some who will disagree with me, no doubt, but I view the tens of thousands of healed bodies, through natural mechanisms, as "empirical evidence" of the efficacy of alternative treatments. I can "directly observe it" – and I have – and the results of this "non-conventional" experiment are highly replicable and repeatable. Actually, as shown through epidemiological studies (previously mentioned), chemotherapy and radiation treatments produce empirical evidence, as well. Over 97% of the time, patients do not last for five years. And this is proven evidence – with no theory or conjecture involved.

When it comes to cancer, you simply desire to be healed. You don't care (largely) how this process takes place; you just want it to happen. Now, if that is truly the case – and it should be – the *proof,* the *empirical evidence,* the ***certifiable healing protocols,*** lie with alternative medicine and treatments, not allopathy. And that statement is nothing but plain, basic, irrefutable truth, based on fact. Take the myth and misconception out of today's treatments for cancer and the effectivity is distilled down to "alternative" treatments alone. And the argument should end there.

As I finish this chapter, I have just received news from a friend about the death of a 32-year old woman acquaintance from breast cancer. We *can* all agree that this is a tragic passing of a mother with two small children – both under four years of age. We *must* all agree that this *has to stop*. Having received an "alternative" protocol that included the alkaline cancer diet and ionized water, her doctor bullied her into abandoning all of this, as it would interfere with her chemotherapy. Sadly, she didn't last long after that oral intervention.

Obviously, not all doctors participate in this type of behavior. Our appeal is that America's physicians will both take the time – and make the effort – to study and understand what God has told us and given to us to strengthen our immune systems and heal our bodies when they become sick or diseased. Doctors are smart people. We can only hope that one day (soon) the forest will become apparent to them through the trees. Our children's lives depend on it.

Note – all testimonies printed as received – with minor corrections for spelling and punctuation.

CHAPTER ELEVEN

"WHAT THE EXPERTS SAY: QUOTES ON CANCER"

"To the cancer establishment, a cancer patient is a profit center. The actual clinical and scientific evidence does not support the claims of the cancer industry. Conventional cancer treatments are in place as the law of the land because they pay, not heal, the best. Decades of the politics-of-cancer-as-usual have kept you from knowing this, and will continue to do so unless you wake up to their reality."

John Diamond, M.D. – Lee Cowden, M.D.

THE certified experts (in my opinion) that are involved in real healing cancer therapies, are those who have a firm grip on – and unbiased understanding of – the cause and effect of this disease and how to, therefore, effectively treat it. Unfortunately (for you and me), most are not found in conventional doctor's offices and hospitals. Many have been driven from the ranks of board certified physicians or ostracized by the very group that is supposed to support them in the healing of cancer patients.

Just what is it that this "alternative" group is telling Americans that has gotten them into so much trouble? What boundaries have they crossed (besides being driven out of the country to Mexico) – which rules have they broken? Why is what they are embracing being suppressed by the mainstream media and the FDA? Who are these heretics, anyway, and what are their crimes? I'm glad you asked.

It is beyond any doubt that these men and women, Ph.D.'s and M.D.'s, Naturopathic and Holistic physicians, nurses, researchers and other alternative health practitioners, are guilty as sin. Against the seemingly wise counsel of conventional medicine, they have dared to use natural medicines, plant extracts, organic supplements, non-synthetic vitamins and minerals, vegan diets, herbs, ionized water, exercise, and many other *unapproved* (and *non-lethal*) methods in an attempt to heal cancer patients without the direct approval of the Food and Drug Administration and the American Medical Association.

How dare they! The nerve of these people – prescribing vitamins and minerals that haven't undergone clinical trials and, thus, remain "unproven." Shame on them! And God Bless them.

While these people may have crossed the allopathic line, they are, in essence and truth, the ***last line of defense*** against a medical consortium that has run amok. Even as I write this, there is a bill in Congress to make all supplements come under the auspices of Pharmaceutical Companies as directed by our friendly Food and Drug Administration. Tell me, why should it be a crime to select and follow your own health care protocol? Why shouldn't I be allowed to make an attempt to heal my cancer using any means that ***I deem*** necessary? Why are doctors not permitted to offer what really works to heal their patients? After all, we've already confessed that doctors are smart people and we need good doctors. Why not allow them to select the treatments and therapies that do the most good for their clientele? Again, what ever happened to "first, do no harm?"

These are questions that beg to be answered. They also long for an adequate explanation of why a patient's right to treatment and a doctor's right to dispense it are not a "freedom" in a free society. What say you? Should it be so? Why can't Joe and Mary treat their five-year-old son who has cancer with diet, good water, and proper supplementation instead of being "forced" to produce him to the local cancer ward for surgery, chemotherapy, and radiation? Where's the choice? Where's this "medical freedom" that we're told we have?

I believe the answer lies within the unvarnished, well-grounded truth about what does – and what does not – work for cancer patients. But it goes deeper than that. Until, and unless, the American public comes to grips with the certain and genuine facts about cancer and its treatments, the status quo, representing the miserable failure that is our cancer industry, will continue. The promises of a "cure" will never be realized, but echoes of assurances concerning new technologies, genetic advancements, and better drugs will bounce off the walls of conventional academia and give "hope" to the masses where, in fact, there is none – when nothing ever changes.

No, until we are ready to call a spade a spade, to demand from the "powers that be" an actual solution to this real problem, to rise up and rage against the machine that is producing no answers to cancer, things will not change and we will continue our march through the doctor's offices, hospitals, and hospice care to the cemeteries and crematoriums that have claimed so many of us – so prematurely.

Only we can alter this state of affairs – and we must be educated and willing to do so. Seek the truth about cancer and what heals it – not what is convenient. That's exactly what the following people have done. They have collectively shouted, "Hey, wait a minute. Something's not right here." And they have sought to make a difference for the sake of their friends, relatives, children, acquaintances, and their patients.

In my humble opinion, these are the real experts. Herein is a representation of those who saw that something was wrong and proceeded on a quest to find the real facts about cancer and what heals it. Many are doctors who discovered that traditional methods were not helping their patients. Some resolved their own cancer issues with "alternative" measures. Most believe that by doing the "same old things – you get the same old results."

All know that cancer is healable, but surgery, chemotherapy, and radiation play little or no role in that process. You be the judge.

Dr. Julian Whitaker is the Director and Founder of the Whitaker Wellness Institute and also the author of the *Whitaker Health and Healing Newsletter*. Following is a statement from his newsletter:

"You must remember this. If you or a loved one ever faces the scourge of cancer, it is *your* life that is at stake, not your doctor's. It's up to you to take control of your own health."

In Dr. Whitaker's small pamphlet, *What I Would Do if I Had Cancer*, the Doctor continues with this:

"Conventional treatment for cancer is based on a faulty paradigm – that the body must be purged of cancer by aggressive and toxic methods such as surgery, chemotherapy and radiation therapy. This seemed reasonable back in 1894 when William Halsted, M.D., did the first radical mastectomy, but it has proven to be so wrong over the last 50 years that continuing to adhere to it constitutes more fraud than honest mistake. Yet, this paradigm dominates conventional cancer therapy. Conventional cancer therapy is toxic and dehumanizing, and it doesn't work. If it did, we wouldn't fear cancer. But people rush into these therapies that don't work because they are too scared to do anything else."

Dr. Bruce West is the founder of Health Alert/Immune Systems, Inc., and the author of the *Health Alert* Newsletter. Health Alert has an advisory board of 10 Medical Doctors and 37 other medical experts from virtually every health field. Dr. West is said by his contemporaries to have treated and healed more heart patients than any other doctor, alive or dead. Here's what he says about cancer and its treatment:

"Cancer is a **systemic** (throughout the body) disease, no matter what your doctor tells you. Telling patients, based on post-operation scans, that 'we got it all' is always a lie. Scans to predict if you are cancer-free are useless. Most cancers have been growing and spreading for 5 to 10 years before they are detected and diagnosed. Billions of cancer cells must be present to show up on any scan. Surgery, although often needed, can spread cancer. The word 'cure' in oncology (cancer care) circles has up to fifty different definitions. The only real cure is the one where you live long enough to die from something other than cancer. These survivors are strong, and most utilize a protocol to treat cancer **everywhere** in their body, rather than relying solely on local surgery, local radiation, and/or chemotherapy."

Dr. Philip Binzel, M.D., was a small town doctor and a graduate of St. Louis University School of Medicine. Dr. Binzel promoted nutritional therapies and laetrile for over 30 years and his success record was outstanding. From his Book, *Alive and Well*, Chapter 14, comes the following exceptional, explanatory information:

"When a patient is found to have a tumor, the only thing the doctor discusses with the patient is what he intends to do about the tumor. If a patient with a tumor is receiving radiation or chemotherapy, the only question that is asked is, 'How is the tumor doing?' No one ever asks how the patient is doing. In my medical training, I remember well seeing patients who were getting radiation and/or chemotherapy. The tumor would get smaller and smaller, but the patient would be getting sicker and sicker. At autopsy we would hear, 'Isn't that marvelous! The tumor is gone!' Yes, it was, but so was the patient. How many millions of times are we going to have to repeat these scenarios before we realize that we are treating the wrong thing?

"In primary cancer, with only a few exceptions, the tumor is neither health-endangering nor life-threatening. What is health-endangering and life-threatening is the spread of that disease through the rest of the body.

"There is nothing in surgery that will prevent the spread of cancer. There is nothing in radiation that will prevent the spread of the disease. There is nothing in chemotherapy that will prevent the spread of the disease. How do we know? Just look at the statistics! There is a statistic known as 'survival time.' Survival time is defined as that interval of time between when the diagnosis is first made in a given patient and when that patient dies from his disease.

"In the past fifty years, tremendous progress has been made in the early diagnosis of cancer. In that period of time, tremendous progress has been made in the surgical ability to remove tumors. Tremendous progress has been made in the use of radiation and chemotherapy in their ability to shrink or destroy tumors. But, the survival time of the cancer patient today is no greater than it was fifty years ago. What does this mean? It obviously means that we are treating the wrong thing!

"The only thing known to mankind today that will prevent the spread of cancer within the body is for that body's own defense mechanisms to once again function normally. That's what nutritional therapy does. It treats the defense mechanism, not the tumor."

Well said, Dr. Binzel. Fact, not fiction, based upon years of study and treating patients. Must be more of that "empirical evidence" stuff.

Dr. Jonathan Wright is the Medical Director of the Tahoma Clinic, located about 20 minutes from downtown Seattle. For over 25 years, this

Clinic has utilized, almost exclusively, preventative medicine and natural treatments with its patients. Dr. Wright is well known for promoting natural supplements over dangerous drugs. The Tahoma Clinic was shut down at gunpoint by federal agents and local police in 1992 for forwarding this "natural treatment" philosophy and for allegedly prescribing unapproved drugs and treatments (natural supplements and vitamins) for sick patients. His offices were ransacked and records were carted off. Over time, he was vindicated. Dr. Wright graduated from Harvard at age 20 and the University of Michigan Medical School at age 24. I told you that doctors were smart.

Dr. Wright says that, ultimately, alternative medicine will flourish – and here's his reasoning:

"It's because it works; it's as simple as that. We may not always understand why or how it works, but the tremendous public groundswell for natural medicine is because people know their own bodies, and they know that it works."

Dr. Wright's quote was taken from an interview with the *Seattle Times* and reported in the July 4, 1995, issue by Danny Westneat.

Dr. Gary Null has a Ph.D. in human nutrition and public health science, and is said by many to be America's leading health and nutrition expert. In his published research entitled, *Death By Medicine*, with Carolyn Dean, M.D., N.D; Martin Feldman, M.D; Debora Rasio, M.D; and Dorothy Smith, Ph.D; Dr. Null expresses the following:

"The FDA continues to interfere with those who offer natural products that compete with prescription drugs. These attacks against natural medicine obscure a lethal problem that, until now, was buried in thousands of pages of scientific text. In response to these baseless challenges to natural medicine, the Nutrition

Institute of America commissioned an independent review of the quality of 'government-approved' medicine. The startling findings from this meticulous study indicate that conventional medicine is *the leading cause of death'* in the United States."

Who would have believed it? But it's absolutely true. Other epidemiological studies show iatrogenics (death by doctor, drugs, hospital) to be the third leading cause of death today in the United States. Actually, when all of the facts and figures are taken into consideration, as Dr. Null illustrates, the cheerleaders for iatrocide are yelling "We're Number One!" And when it comes to cancer, many of the hundreds of thousands of death certificates that aren't attributed to this disease – and should be – state that the patient died of pneumonia, liver disease, heart failure (brought on by chemotherapeutic agents), or some other malady that was a result of the **cancer treatment!** Here, let me juggle those statistics for you.

Thank you Dr. Null for your continued diligence in forwarding natural medicine and exposure of the truth surrounding iatrogenesis and "death by medicine." And my support is not designed to slam our doctors. No, it is simply meant to show that we have a severe problem when it comes to healthcare, especially cancer care, and we need to do something about it. Now.

Dr. Hiromi Shinya is the Chief of Surgical Endoscopy at Beth Israel Medical Center and Clinical Professor of Surgery at the Albert Einstein College of Medicine. Dr. Shinya has done over 370,000 colonoscopies and co-invented the "polyp removal" tool for this procedure. The following quotes are from a June 27th, 2009, lecture by Dr. Shinya:

"Daily consumption of beef will inevitably produce prostate problems and cancer.

"Vegetable proteins *'freeze'* cancer cells.

"Meat protein, and especially casein (protein from milk), stimulate and fertilize cancer growth.

"The increased hormones in milk cause breast cancer, as well as prostate and infertility problems."

Do you think that the good doctor promotes meat and milk? Not! Read *The China Study*, by T. Colin Campbell, and you will see the complete documentation about how cancer, meat, and milk are directly related. Dr. Shinya has seen more than enough colons and colon cancer to understand the connection between diet and this disease. He recommends Kangen Water™ to his patients and has seen a "zero percent" recurrence of any kind of cancer when his patients follow his prescribed lifestyle, including drinking Kangen Water™.

Dr. T. Colin Campbell, with his son Tom, co-authored the most comprehensive study of health and nutrition ever conducted, the previously mentioned, *The China Study*. Dr. Campbell has authored more than 300 research papers and is Jacob Gould Schurman Professor Emeritus of Nutritional Biochemistry at Cornell University. *The China Study* was the result and culmination of a twenty-year partnership involving Cornell University, Oxford University, and the Chinese Academy of Preventive Medicine. After reading this book, one clearly understands that the results of this amazing study are entrenched in pure science. And the message is this: Change your diet and you will dramatically reduce your risk of cancer, heart disease, diabetes and obesity.

On page 317 of this tediously documented scientific work, Dr. Campbell makes this statement:

"Our tax dollars are used to make the pharmaceutical industry more profitable. One could argue that this is justified by gains in public health, but the alarming fact is that this litany of research into drugs, genes, devices and technology research *will never cure our chronic diseases*. Our chronic diseases are largely the result of infinitely complex assaults on our bodies resulting from eating bad food. No single chemical intervention will ever equal the power of consuming the healthiest food. In addition, isolated chemicals in drug form can be very dangerous. The National Cancer Institute itself states, 'What is clear is that most of our current treatments will produce some measure of adversity.' There is no danger to eating a healthy diet, and there are far more benefits, including massive cost savings both on the front end of preventing disease and on the back end of treating disease. So, why is our government ignoring the abundant scientific research supporting a dietary approach in favor of largely ineffective, potentially dangerous drug and device interventions?"

Good question, Doc. Notice the words "abundant scientific research." The research is there; the results are in; the conclusions are factual and specific. With general health or disease, especially cancer, diet works – drugs don't.

G. Edward Griffin is not a doctor. Rather, he is a documentary film producer, writer, lecturer, and was formerly a child actor. Ed is well known for his literary exposés on the United Nations and the Federal Reserve. More notably, however, and of extreme importance to cancer sufferers, Mr. Griffin is the author of *World Without Cancer*, the narrative history of vitamin B-17. What is astonishing is that the book is still in print today, even though it was originally published back in 1974. In at least its 15th printing, and having been updated, this work is as relevant today as it was over three decades ago. Mr. Griffin dedicates his book to "the millions of cancer victims and their loved ones whose suffering has been the tragic cost of scientific arrogance and political vested interest."

World Without Cancer is the story of Laetrile, commonly called amygdalin or vitamin B-17. While it is indeed a story, it is not a novel. Based upon volumes and volumes of research, this factual presentation brings to light the true history of an anti-cancer, natural substance that many say "cures" cancer. The history of Laetrile treatment for cancer and the science behind it date back to the early 20th Century and have been proven and documented beyond any doubt. I highly recommend that you read this book. Following is an interesting tidbit from Mr. Griffin's masterpiece (Page 151):

"As we have seen, however, the health records of the Hunzakuts and Eskimos, and many other groups around the world, are statistically conclusive that vitamin B-17 does control cancer in human beings with an effectiveness approaching 100%. There can be little controversy over that. But what about cancer once it already has started? Can B-17 restore a person to health after he has contracted the disease?

"The answer is yes, *if* it is caught in time, and *if* the patient is not too badly damaged by prior X-ray treatment or toxic drugs. Unfortunately, most cancer victims start taking Laetrile only after their disease is so far advanced that they have been given up as hopeless by routine medical channels. Usually, they have been told that they have only a few more months or weeks to live. And it is in this tragic state of near death that they turn to vitamin therapy as a last resort. If they die – and, indeed, many of them do – then they are counted as statistical failures for Laetrile. In reality, it is a victory for Laetrile that *any* of them should be saved at this stage. For, once a deficiency disease has progressed so far, the damage it does simply cannot be reversed."

It is very unfortunate that most cancer sufferers who turn to alternative therapies do so after having undergone significant conventional treatments. And, sadly, most are left in the deteriorated physical condition that Ed Griffin describes above. Because of immune killing drugs and radiotherapy, many are near death and arrive too late for "alternatives" to help them.

Sandra Olson has a Master's Degree in Education and has been teaching the "Budwig protocol" to thousands of eager listeners over the past 4-5 years. While not a doctor, she has been able to witness the amazing recovery of those cancer patients who chose to utilize the flax oil/cottage cheese diet promoted by Dr. Johanna Budwig. Below are a few paragraphs from an article that Ms. Olson published and submitted to the ezinearticles.com website and is also found on her site at www.Budwig-videos.com:

> "As moderator of a large Budwig discussion group, I've answered hundreds of questions and have worked with many people who have overcome cancer. For example, Peter was given only months to live when he was diagnosed with liver cancer. He had two tumors that were growing steadily. He refused conventional treatment and began the Budwig protocol. Once he worked all parts of the plan into his daily routine, the tumors began to diminish and were negligible in three months. A year and a half later he remains cancer free. His doctor is amazed.

> "Janice had breast cancer with metastasis to the bones in her spine. Her arms were so swollen that she couldn't fully raise them. She chose the Budwig protocol instead of conventional treatment. After a few months, her arms returned to normal and the cancer was gone. She now leads a very active life.

> "One man had multiple myeloma and went through every treatment a top U.S. clinic has to offer. After a year of terrible side effects from chemo, radiation, etc., his doctors said he had only weeks to live. His wife then found the Budwig plan and started

him on it. He slowly improved and after six months was declared cancer-free by the doctors who had previously said he was terminal.

"A prostate cancer patient was given six months to live when he was diagnosed at age 69. He began the Budwig diet and lived well to age 85.

"There are many more true experiences like these from people who had various kinds of cancer or arthritis, asthma or diabetes, as well as other ailments. The Budwig diet and protocol can help to overcome disease as well as prevent disease through healthful nutrition and lifestyle. It's life-changing information."

Many in conventional research and medicine will pass off this data and these testimonies as not being viable proof since the information was not collected in a clinical environment. I can tell you for sure, however, that those who have survived cancer by using the Budwig protocol would give them a great argument on this subject – especially since traditional therapies failed most of them.

Yes, I know. It's only cottage cheese and flax oil. But the years of scientific study and volumes of documentation supporting this synergistic combination of sufurated proteins and omega fatty acids, and demonstration of how the concoction works for cancer patients, was ***proven beyond any doubt*** over seven decades ago. And it is as effective today as it was then. Many will testify to that fact.

Wade Lightheart is the founder of the Institute for Advanced Natural Health Sciences and a world champion body builder. He is what I would call an "extreme" advocate of personal nutrition and holistic health practitioners. He has proven the power of good nutrition and water through his own life and forwards his health philosophy and lifestyle protocol via his A.W.E.S.O.M.E. program; air, water, exercise, sunlight, optimizers (enzymes, probiotics, amino acids, minerals, vitamins), mental beliefs and attitudes, and education. I've had the pleasure of speaking with Wade on several occasions. Let's listen to him for a moment:

> "You see, doctors study pathologies and seek out methods to eradicate the symptoms of a disease – which is one way to deal with the symptoms. However, after witnessing my sister and countless other individuals endure the horrors of chemotherapy, radiation, and bone marrow transplants, this approach didn't make sense. Think about it. If you wanted to become healthier, would you go take a round of chemotherapy? Or subject yourself to high levels of radiation? If you simply stop and ask yourself, 'Does this make sense?' – you tend to get clarity around a problem. It's for this reason that I chose to study EXCELLENCE through optimizing cellular functioning through manipulation of the factors that make your cell work properly. If a cell is working the way nature intended, it's reasonable to assume a person would be less likely to develop cancer or to overcome the disease if they already have it."

Wade is also a great supporter of ionized water and promotes it along with exercise, diet, and a healthy lifestyle.

Mike Vrentas is the Vice President of the Independent Cancer Research Foundation (ICRF) and was mentioned as a "cancer coach" in a previous chapter. Simply put, when it comes to cancer, Mike knows what works. I sat down with Mike in his home recently. He has an excellent understanding of the cancer process and what to do to heal it. In his own words:

> "I have spent the past ten years and thousands of hours (along with my wife) researching 'gentle', alternative treatments for cancer and chronic disease. This does not include drugs, chemotherapy

or radiation, but gentle treatments of rebuilding your body by re-balancing the inner terrain so the cancer cannot survive.

"A very good comparison would be a swimming pool. When the pH drops in the water of a swimming pool and the chemicals become out of balance, this causes algae to grow out of control. In the swimming pool you raise the pH in the water and re-balance the chemicals. The algae then die, dropping to the bottom of the pool, where it's vacuumed out, and one has a nice clean pool. It's very similar with cancer.

"In the event of cancer, the pH has dropped in your bodily fluids and within the inner terrain of your body. Cancer is a nutritional deficiency of the autonomic nervous system and cells, and the inability of the pancreas to produce enough enzymes to dissolve the foreign masses, which grow in each of our bodies daily. This nutritional imbalance allows the amino acids and hormones to get out of balance, which, in turn, causes a domino effect, damaging the DNA inside the cells.

"To win the battle with cancer and chronic disease, you must raise the pH of your bodily fluids from that of acidic to slightly alkaline (7.345) and re-balance the inner terrain of your body – just as in the swimming pool. This is done with a change of diet and lifestyle. For example, this protocol would include detoxing the body, consumption of fruits and vegetables, juicing, nutritional supplementation, the addition of electron-rich unsaturated fats combined with a sulfur protein (Budwig protocol), and vitamin and mineral supplements. With the addition of this type of a regimen, the cancer cannot survive and starts to die, the same as the algae in the swimming pool."

Dr. A. True Ott, PhD., is the author of *Wellness Secrets For Life, An Owner's Manual for the Human Body.* Dr. Ott promotes the necessity of minerals and water for the proper functioning of the body's muscles, nerves, blood vessels and organs. He understands the results of ingesting sodium fluoride, especially in soda pop and toothpaste. From the referenced book:

"Mothers, if your little ones are having trouble concentrating at home or in school, or have been diagnosed as 'attention deficit' – perhaps you would be well advised to look for the culprit (and the solution to the problem) no further than your home medicine cabinet (your tube of toothpaste) and your friendly neighborhood school's water fountain!!

"How does sodium fluoride kill rats? Are you sure you want to know? When sodium fluoride enters your stomach, it reacts with your stomach acid and changes into yet another NEW inorganic compound called fluoric acid. Fluoric acid can be purchased over the counter in most hardware and grocery stores for removing rust stains from your clothing. It is a reverse, or 'backwards' acid because it will not melt your clothing and it will not even bother your skin. BUT YET IT WILL DISSOLVE GLASS UPON CONTACT. ATTENTION – sodium fluoride inhibits over 100 critically important enzyme functions in the human body and is directly attributed to over 50,000 cancer deaths each year. The main function of sodium fluoride when used as a rat poison is TO DESTROY ENZYME FUNCTION. This causes the rat to starve to death while eating all the food it desires. This is called death by malnutrition. As fluoride levels increase, the ability of the body to get adequate nutrition decreases by the lack of enzyme functions. Sodium Fluoride also disrupts DNA repair, causes genetic damage, and increases the risk of hereditary cancers, and directly accelerates the aging process."

I told you so.

Webster Kehr, better known as the **"Cancer Tutor"**, is probably one of the most knowledgeable researchers in the alternative, anti-cancer movement. The Cancer Tutor website boasts the most complete information on cancer and its treatments and is a virtual library of data on a multitude of anti-cancer disciplines, from cause to cure. Find it at www. cancertutor.com. Webster is President of the Independent Cancer Research Foundation and an author of many white papers and ebooks on cancer, physics and mathematics. I consider him a personal friend and met with him for a couple of days on a recent trip to the Midwest. Although there are literally volumes of quotable data and information that I have gleaned from him in person and on his website, I will quote herein one short story and you can visit his site for the rest:

"Suppose you own an antique dining room table which is worth many tens of thousands of dollars. Suppose your butler tells you that there are dozens of cockroaches crawling around on your priceless table and you will be having dinner guests in one hour.

"Your butler informs you that his job description does not include killing cockroaches and, as he is leaving your house, he offers you four options for getting rid of the cockroaches:

1) He offers you a chainsaw to 'slash' the little critters to pieces,
2) He offers you a large and powerful flamethrower to 'burn' the critters to pieces,
3) He offers you two gallons of a highly toxic liquid chemical to 'poison' the critters, and
4) He offers you an old $1 flyswatter.

"Which of the four options would you use to get rid of the cockroaches? Would you choose one of the first three options (slash, burn, and poison) because they are highly potent at killing cockroaches, or would you choose the cheap, wimpy flyswatter?

"Think about why you would make your choice.

"Most likely you would pick the flyswatter because the other three items (which are far more powerful than a flyswatter at killing cockroaches) are also massively powerful *at destroying* your priceless table!!

"Chemotherapy (the toxic chemical above), surgery (the chainsaw above), and radiation (the flamethrower above) do kill cancer cells, but they also kill healthy cells (the priceless antique table), damage the immune system, damage the ability of your digestive tract to process nutrients, etc., *because they do not target cancer cells*. Thus, these treatments cannot cure cancer (which has spread) without killing the patient first.

"By comparison, alternative cancer treatments (the flyswatter), while *not as powerful* as the other items, are *far more effective* at treating cancer because these treatments *either target cancer cells or do not damage your healthy cells*. Thus, they can be given in *much higher doses* than any of the "orthodox" cancer treatments. Plus, the many alternative cancer treatments can generally be combined.

"A person can drink a quart of carrot juice but they cannot drink a quart of chemotherapy."

Bill Henderson was introduced as a cancer coach in a previous chapter and is publisher of one of the best anti-cancer newsletters available. Again, do consider using his services if you are stricken with cancer, and subscribe to his monthly missive – it's free. Bill is a proponent of immune building supplements and in his book, *Cancer Free*, he answers the question about why these are a first priority (page 92):

"Taking appropriate immune system boosting products will almost certainly insure that your cancer will not recur. Without this treatment, continued after you are declared 'cancer-free,' your cancer will almost certainly recur months or years after completion of your 'debulking' therapy.

"No instruments or tests today can detect the relatively small number of cancer cells that *always remain* after conventional treatment. Those cells are, by definition, the *hardiest*. With your immune system *destroyed by the chemotherapy*, radiation or surgery, they continue to divide in a *'cancer friendly'* environment.

"If you or a loved one is diagnosed with cancer, immune system boosting is *PRIORITY ONE*. Best of all, this treatment is what is known as an *'adjunctive'* therapy. That means it does not require you to challenge your cancer doctor to approve an 'alternative' treatment. With enough study of the available research, almost any respectable doctor should cheer you on in your use of these products. If he or she does not, *take them anyway*, and consider finding another doctor."

You've got to like that last sentence. Pretty bold of Bill. But when you are steeped in truth, you just have to let people know.

Dr. Andrew Weil, M.D., really needs no introduction. He is a graduate of Harvard Medical School, and has worked for both the National Institute of Mental Health and the Harvard Botanical Museum. He has extensively studied plants and their healing properties. Dr. Weil is the founder of the Arizona Center for Integrative Medicine and is considered to be (by his peers) one of the world's leaders in integrative medicine. In his sixth book, *Spontaneous Healing*, released in 1995, Dr. Weil states the following regarding cancer:

> "Current therapies for cancer, both conventional and alternative, are far from satisfactory. Conventional medicine has three main treatments: surgery, radiation, and chemotherapy, of which only the first makes sense. If cancer is in one location only and accessible to a surgeon's knife, it can be excised and eliminated permanently. Unfortunately, only a small percentage of cancers meet those criteria, principally cancers of the skin and uterine cervix. In far too many cases cancer has already spread to more than one site by the time of its discovery or is somewhere in the body that is beyond the reach of a surgical cure.
>
> "Radiation and chemotherapy are crude treatments that will be obsolete before long. If you have cancer and are faced with a decision about whether to use conventional therapies, the question you must try to answer is this: Will the damage done to the cancer justify the damage done to the immune system?"

I find most interesting the comment about chemotherapy and radiation being obsolete before long. While we can only hope that this is true, it has been sixteen years since the release of this book. Hopefully, most of us will live to see the demise of these barbaric treatments. Unfortunately, many cancer sufferers will not.

Ty Bollinger has produced one of the best and most usable books ever written about cancer. Many of Ty's family members died of cancer. He, like most of the rest of us, asked "why?" His question, and subsequent research, led him to the truth about this disease and produced his excellent exposé entitled *Cancer – Step Outside The Box*, first published in 2006, and now in at least its third printing. While there's a ton of good "meat" in this book, I believe that the link between cancer and root canal dentistry needs a little more exposure. Ty quotes an actual dentist, Dr. Hal Huggins, who is a leader in "biological dentistry" in this excerpt, page 340, from his book:

"In 1993, Dr. Hal Huggins, D.D.S., gave a lecture to the Cancer Control Society. In an almost comical fashion, Dr. Huggins stated, *'Then we get into the root canal business, and that is the most tragic of all. Isn't there something you can put in the center of the canal that is safe? Yeah, there probably is, but that is not where the problem is.* **The problem with a root canal is that it is dead.** *Let's equate that. Let's say you have got a ruptured appendix, so you go to the phone book, and who do you look up? Let's see, we have a surgeon and a taxidermist, who do you call? You going to get it bronzed? That is all we do to a dead tooth. We put a gold crown on it, looks like it has been bronzed. It doesn't really matter what you embalm the dead tooth with, it is still dead, and within that dead tooth we have bacteria, and these bacteria are in the absence of oxygen. In the absence of oxygen most things die except bacteria. They undergo something called a* **pleomorphic** *change...like a mutation...they learn to live in the absence of oxygen...and now produce* **thio-ethers**, *some of the strongest poisons on the planet that are not radioactive.'"*

If you recall, we have addressed root canals and their very possible link to cancer – especially breast cancer. Please, pay attention to this one. Many thanks to Ty and Doc Huggins.

Dr. Robert O. Young, Ph.D., has degrees in nutrition, chemistry, and microbiology and has researched mycotic infections (yeast, mold, fungus) and their relationship to disease for many years. He is currently vice president of research and development for InnerLight International and author of *The pH Miracle: Balance Your Diet, Reclaim Your Health*. Dr. Young is a promoter of an alkaline diet and believes that acidity is a major cause of sickness and disease. In his white paper entitled, *Overacidity and*

Overgrowth of Yeast, Fungus and Moulds, Dr. Young has this to say about cancer, hormones and acidity:

> "Cancer is not a virus; it is an acid problem produced by a mould. It is an infection due to excess fermentation in the weakest parts of the body. What causes cancer in cigarettes is the yeast and sugar they use to accelerate the fermentation process in the tobacco leaves. Cancer is not a localized problem that is metastasizing. Cancer is a systemic problem that has localized. We know through research that the supplementation of hormones can be a risk factor for breast cancer. When you supplement hormones, those hormones are subject to fermentation in a body that is out of balance, and when hormones are fermented, they produce an acid, which has to be eliminated. These acids are then stored in areas of fatty tissue and what more perfect place to put it than the breast. How can emotion or fear cause rotting processes? Biologically, it's simple. Emotions create acidity through the release of hormones that are then fermented, which produces the acid. And, we then start craving the foods we should basically avoid."

Sugar, acid, fermentation – the buzzwords that are always linked to cancer. Remember, cancer cells are anaerobic (without oxygen) and feed by fermenting sugar in an acid environment.

The following are "snap-shot" quotes from doctors and oncologists – some questioning their own profession, others expounding upon the cause and the cure – all waxing philosophically about the truth (please give these some considerable thought):

My take is that oncologist **James F. Holland, M.D.**, had pretty much reached the tipping point when he said the following in *The Krebiozen Story*:

"My definition of cancer quackery is the deliberate misapplication of a diagnostic or treatment procedure in a patient with cancer... The culprit who victimizes his fellow man suffering from cancer... all the while greedily enriching himself, is a quack, a criminal, a jackal among men who deserves the scorn and ostracism of society. Because human life is at stake, he must be controlled."

Katy bar the door! What do you really think, Doc? Isn't it refreshing coming from a doctor and oncologist?

Dr. Glen Warner, M.D., and another oncologist, adds his two-bits worth to the chemo deception:

"Chemotherapy is an incredibly lucrative business for doctors, hospitals, and pharmaceutical companies. The medical establishment wants everyone to follow the same exact protocol. They don't want to see the chemotherapy industry go under, and that's the number one obstacle to any progress in oncology."

Dr. William Campbell Douglass, M.D., shoots straight from the hip regarding radiation scans and cancer:

"Studies have found that one percent of all new cancers are caused by CT scans alone. In fact, mainstream researchers have estimated that CT scans performed just in 2007 – just that one single year – will eventually lead to 29,000 cancers. No matter how you look at it, radiation-based tests come with major risks – and studies have found that half of them are completely unnecessary, and many more are wildly redundant. I won't say never, ever get an X-ray or CT scan – but before you put yourself into a lead-lined tube, make sure it's really necessary."

Dr. Leonard Coldwell, N.D., world-renowned Naturopathic Doctor and author, challenges us to look inside ourselves when it comes to cancer:

"All illnesses are caused by a direct violation of God's or Nature's laws. It is a violation of the use of power and free will that you have. It is an imbalanced energy system that causes your immune system to fail. It is self-neglect, self-denial, self-hatred, or subconscious suicide that leads to cancer. It's you!"

Can't be me, Doc! Let's see – who can I blame?

This section would not be complete without a quotation from **Mike Adams, the renowned "Health Ranger,"** and an invitation to enjoy his short missive entitled, *Welcome to the Town of Allopath*. This "politically incorrect" but very accurate fable is an illustrative exposé of conventional medicine, pharmaceutical companies, and the FDA. Initially, I wanted to just mention the website where all could find it but, knowing that many folks who are reading this book do not have computer access, I felt it necessary to reprint it right here – of course – with the permission of the author. I guarantee that you are going to like it. So fasten your seatbelt, put your seatback in an upright position, and enjoy your short journey to the town of "*Allopath*":

"There once was a town called Allopath. It had many people, streets and cars, but, due to budget limitations, there were no stop signs or traffic lights anywhere in Allopath.

"Not surprisingly, traffic accidents were common. Cars would crash into each other at nearly every intersection. But business was booming for the auto repair shops and local hospitals, which dominated the economy of Allopath.

"As the population of Allopath grew, traffic accidents increased to an alarming level. Out of desperation, the city council hired Doctor West, a doctor of the Motor Division (M.D.) to find a solution.

"Dr. West spent days examining traffic accidents. He carried an assortment of technical gear – microscopes, chemical analysis equipment, lab gear – and put them all to work as part of his investigation. The townspeople of Allopath watched on with great curiosity while Dr. West went about his work, meticulously documenting and analyzing each traffic accident, and they awaited his final report with great interest.

"After weeks of investigation, Dr. West called the people of Allopath to a town meeting for the release of his report. There, in front of the city council and most of the residents of Allopath, he announced his findings: 'Traffic accidents are caused by skid marks.'

"As Dr. West explained, he found and documented a near-100% correlation between traffic accidents and skid marks. 'Wherever we find these cars colliding,' he explained, 'we also find these skid marks.'

"The town had 'Skid Marks Disease,' the doctor explained, and the answer to the town's epidemic of traffic accidents would 'require nothing more than treating Skid Marks Disease by making the streets skid-proof,' Dr. West exclaimed, to great applause from the townspeople.

"The city paid Dr. West his consulting fee, then asked the good doctor to propose a method for treating this Skid Marks Disease. As chance would have it, Dr. West had recently been on a trip to Hawaii paid for by a chemical company that manufactured roadaceuticals; special chemicals used to treat roads for situations just like this one. He recommended a particular chemical coating to the city council: teflon.

"'We can treat this Skid Marks Disease by coating the roads with teflon,' Dr. West explained. 'The streets will then be skid-proof, and all the traffic accidents will cease!' He went on to describe the physical properties of teflon and how its near-frictionless coating would deter nearly all vehicle skids.

"The city council heartily agreed with Dr. West, and they issued new public bonds to raise the money required to buy enough teflon to coat all the city's streets. Within weeks, the streets were completely coated, and the skid marks all but disappeared.

"The city council paid Dr. West another consulting fee and thanked him for his expertise. The problem of traffic accidents in Allopath was solved, they thought. Although the cure was expensive, they were convinced it was worth it.

"But things weren't well in Allopath. Traffic accidents quadrupled. Hospital beds were overflowing with injured residents. Auto repair businesses were booming so much that most of the city council members decided to either open their own car repair shops or invest in existing ones.

"Week after week, more and more residents of Allopath were injured, and their cars were repeatedly damaged. Money piled into the pockets of the car repair shops, hospitals, tow truck companies and car parts retailers.

"The town economic advisor, observing this sharp increase in economic activity, announced that Allopath was booming. Its economy was healthier than ever, and Allopath could look forward to a great year of economic prosperity!

"There were jobs to be had at the car repair shops. There were more nurses needed at the hospital. 'Help wanted' signs appeared all over town – at the paramedic station, the tow truck shops, and the auto glass businesses. Unemployment dropped to near zero.

"But the traffic accidents continued to increase. And yet there were no skid marks.

"The city council was baffled. They thought they had solved the problem. Skid Marks Disease had been eradicated by the teflon treatment. Why were traffic accidents still happening?

"They called a town meeting to discuss the problem, and following a short discussion of the problem, an old hermit, who lived in the forest just outside of Allopath, addressed the townspeople. 'There is no such thing as Skid Marks Disease,' he explained. 'This disease was invented by the roadaceuticals company to sell you teflon coatings.'

"The townspeople were horrified to hear such a statement. They knew Skid Marks Disease existed. The doctor had told them so. How could this hermit, who had no Motor Division (M.D.) degree, dare tell them otherwise? How could he question their collective town wisdom in such a way?

"'This is a simple problem,' the hermit continued. 'All we need to do is build stop signs and traffic lights. Then the traffic accidents will cease.'

"Without pause, one city council member remarked, 'But how

can we afford stop signs? We've spent all our money on teflon treatments!'

"The townspeople agreed. They had no money to buy stop signs.

"Another council member added, 'And how can we stop anyway? The streets are all coated with teflon. If we build stop signs, we'll waste all the money we've spent on teflon!'

"The townspeople agreed, again. What use were stop signs if they couldn't stop their cars anyway?

"The hermit replied, 'But the stop signs will eliminate the need for teflon. People will be able to stop their cars, and accidents will cease. The solution is simple.'

"But what might happen if stop signs actually worked, the townspeople wondered. How would it affect the booming economy of Allopath? Realizing the consequences, a burly old man who owned a local repair shop jumped to his feet and said, 'If we build these stop signs, and traffic accidents go down, I'll have to fire most of my workers!'

"It was at that moment that most of the townspeople realized there own jobs were at stake. If stop signs were built, nearly everyone would be unemployed. They all had jobs in emergency response services, car repair shops, hospitals and teflon coating maintenance. Some were now sales representatives of the roadaceuticals company. Others were importers of glass, tires, steel and other parts for cars. A few clever people were making a fortune selling wheelchairs and crutches to accident victims.

"One enterprising young gentleman started a scientific journal that published research papers describing all the different kinds of Skid Marks Diseases that had been observed and documented. Another person, a fitness enthusiast, organized an annual run to raise funds to find the cure for Skid Marks Disease. It was a popular event, and all the townspeople participated as best they could: jogging, walking, or just pushing themselves along in their wheelchairs.

"One way or another, nearly everyone in Allopath was economically tied to Skid Marks Disease.

"Out of fear of losing this economic prosperity, the townspeople voted to create a new public safety agency: the Frequent Drivers Association (FDA). This FDA would be responsible for approving or rejecting all signage, technology and chemical coatings related to the town's roads.

"The FDA's board members were chosen from among the business leaders of the community: the owner of the car shop, the owner of the ambulance company, and of course, Dr. West.

"Soon after its inception, the FDA announced that Skid Marks Disease was, indeed, very real, as it had been carefully documented by a doctor and recently published in the town Skid Marks Disease journal. Since there were no studies whatsoever showing stop signs to be effective for reducing traffic accidents, the FDA announced that stop signs were to be outlawed, and that any person attempting to sell stop signs would be charged with fraud and locked up in the town jail.

"This pleased the townspeople of Allopath. With the FDA, they knew their jobs were safe. They could go on living their lives of economic prosperity, with secure jobs, knowing that the FDA would outlaw any attempt to take away their livelihood. They still had a lot of traffic accidents, but at least their jobs were secure.

"And so life continued in Allopath. For a short while, at least. As traffic accidents continued at a devastating rate, more and more residents of Allopath were injured or killed. Many were left bed-ridden, unable to work, due to their injuries.

"In time, the population dwindled. The once-booming town of Allopath eventually became little more than a ghost town. The hospital closed its doors, the FDA was disbanded, and the Skid Marks Disease journal stopped printing.

"The few residents remaining eventually realized nothing good had come of Skid Marks Disease, the teflon coatings and the FDA. No one was any better off, as all the town's money had been spent on the disease: the teflon coatings, car parts and emergency services. No one was any healthier, or happier, or longer-lived. Most, in fact, had lost their entire families to Skid Marks Disease.

"And the hermit? He continued to live just outside of town, at the end of a winding country road, where he lived a simple life with no cars, no roads, no teflon coatings and no FDA.

"He outlived every single resident of Allopath. He gardened, took long walks through the forest, and gathered roots, leaves and berries to feed himself. In his spare time, he constructed stop signs, waiting for the next population to come along, and hoping they might listen to an old hermit with a crazy idea:

"…that prevention is the answer, not the treatment of symptoms."

What a great job, Mike! We would all be so much better off (and healthier) if we would just be mindful of the "not-so-hidden" message attached to this "not-so-unrealistic" story. As we leave *Allopath* (but not its inherent epistle), let's listen to what Mike has to say about vitamin D and cancer:

"We already know that vitamin D, all by itself, can prevent nearly 4 out of 5 cancers (documentation from the following website (http://www.naturalnews.com/021892.html). It also helps prevent heart disease, diabetes, depression, seasonal flu and kidney disease. Distribute free vitamin D supplements across the entire population and you solve the doctor shortage problem in one year as the public gets healthier and reduces doctor visits.

"It's a simple, cost-effective solution that any intelligent nation would embrace without a second thought: Invest a few pennies in the health of the population and save yourself many dollars in reduced health care costs. Regular vitamin D supplementation has no negative side effects and requires no prescriptions, no injections and no visits to the doctor. What's not to like about that?

"Except the sick care industry doesn't like it at all. Drug companies, hospitals, conventional doctors, med schools, medical journals and now even the mainstream media all generate extreme profits from the ongoing business of sickness and disease. Vitamin D would disrupt their profit agenda and *send people home healthy and well* instead of bringing them back into the hospital sick and diseased.

"America, you see, does not have a *shortage* of doctors…it has an *excess* of disease. And that's an excess that the sick-care system seems determined to continue."

Mike is editor of NaturalNews.com and an expert in health and healing.

Dr. John Bailer, an epidemiologist at Montreal's McGill University, gives us his own statistical analysis of mainstream cancer statistics in the following that was quoted in a 1986 edition of the *New England Journal of Medicine*:

"The five year cancer survival statistics of the American Cancer Society are very misleading. They now count things that are not cancer and, because we are able to diagnose at an earlier stage of the disease, patients falsely appear to live longer. Our whole cancer research in the past 20 years has been a failure. More people over 30 are dying from cancer than ever before…More women with mild or benign diseases are being included in statistics and reported as being 'cured.' When government officials point to survival figures and say they are winning the war against cancer, they are using those survival rates improperly."

Many epidemiologists, researchers, statisticians, and doctors echo these same sentiments regarding the obvious, intentional manipulation of cancer statistics.

Dr. Sherry Rogers, M.D., offers up this next summation regarding the truth surrounding cancer symptoms and causes in her book, *Detoxify or Die*:

"You have been brainwashed into believing that the diagnosis given to your condition, a mere label, is the end of the line. But nothing could be further (and more dangerously) from the truth. In fact, the name or label that has been given to your collection of symptoms is totally inconsequential. The only thing that matters is what has caused the symptoms."

And that's exactly what *you* should be concerned about – that which really *matters.* While mainstream medicine concentrates continuously and exclusively on the symptoms themselves, cancer sufferers should focus on what *caused* these indicators that something was wrong. In other words, resolve the disease – not the symptoms.

Linus Pauling, two-time Nobel Prize winner, said it succinctly and accurately:

"Everyone should know that the 'war on cancer' is largely a fraud."

Here, here.

And, finally, a tell-it-like-it-really-is summation from an oncology nurse that is on the front lines of conventional cancer treatments every day – who I would call the *real* expert – in her own words:

"I have been an oncology nurse for 12 years now. My first 3 years of that were spent in a large city's pediatric bone marrow transplant and oncology unit, followed by nine years in an outpatient adult oncology setting. I have always felt 'called' to work with cancer patients, and feel that I am blessed tremendously by the privilege of caring for this specialty population.

"Among other things, it truly puts life in perspective for me, helping me to value things that really matter – and not getting so upset by the trivial things in life, such as getting stuck in a traffic jam or waiting so long in the grocery store line. And the patients are so appreciative of the care you give them at this extremely difficult time in their lives.

"All this to say that, for the past five years, I have felt a growing angst within me whenever I am at work. You see, the drugs we give the patients in an attempt to 'cure' them (cure, in most cases, meaning a 5-year survival period without the cancer recurring) often do MUCH more harm than good. Side effects include such things as overwhelming fatigue, temporary or permanent loss of feeling in the feet, nausea, skin rashes and burns, loss of appetite and weight…the list could go on and on.

"Frequently, patients will have a week or two in between their chemo and/or radiation treatments and will come to the clinic for follow-up visits on their breaks. When I ask them how they are feeling, they always respond, 'So much better now that I am not receiving the chemo.' My standard response to them without even consciously thinking has been, 'It's amazing how good you feel when we are not poisoning you!' Now, I realize how true that statement is – *we are truly poisoning them in an attempt to make them better!*

"To the best of my knowledge, in no other medical field do we give toxic and damaging drugs to the patient to cure them. If there is a defect in an organ, tissue, muscle, or bone, it is repaired or replaced with a new one. With infection, antibiotics are given to help the body's immune system rid the body of the infection. In cardiac arrest, all efforts are made to help the heart function as it should – through numerous means – none of which are poison!

"So, why then, with cancer, do we use these toxic drugs – drugs that in themselves can cause cancer (I have seen this numerous times in my career – patients receiving chemo and/or radiation will have a new cancer crop up years later as a result of their treatment!)? It is a question that won't be answered until too many people, especially cancer patients, start asking and demanding answers of oncology professionals."

Tina H., Oncology Nurse

I think we all agree, Tina, it's way beyond time to start asking why.

EXPERT – a person with a high degree of skill in or knowledge of a certain subject (www.thefreedictionary.com).

Certainly we can agree that doctors are "experts" when it comes to diagnosis, surgery, and conventional treatments. For the most part, with few exceptions, the majority of us would not argue with this assessment. After all, doctors have worked long and hard to get where they are. Unfortunately (and by their own admission), they have not been trained in nutrition, nor in what causes the immune system to be compromised that, subsequently, allows the onset of cancer in our bodies.

Cancer needs an expert – a master, professional, wizard, crackerjack – a specialist that understands (as much as man can) the wonderful workings of the human body and how these processes labor together to maintain homeostasis, promote both the chemical and electrical interactions of the cells, and heal the physical being, when necessary. As stated, our doctors are not educated in this proficiency as it is not a part of allopathic medicine. Doesn't it make sense, then, to put our "cancerous" bodies into the hands of the real experts – those who have researched and studied the masterful functions within our individual internal environments that allow us to heal, when given the proper ingredients?

I sincerely hope you are saying, "Yeah, when you put it that way – it makes perfect sense." And it does. This is no slam on doctors. Would you hire an electrician to fix your plumbing? A landscaper to remodel your home? A chef to be your mechanic? Probably not. And the reason is basic. You simply want the best trained, most knowledgeable, and most capable – the real expert – to perform those services for you. In the final analysis, you just want it done right and done well.

The same is true with cancer. When you are diagnosed (and almost half of Americans will be), you just want to get well. And now you know that, beyond any reasonable doubt, your best shot is with the "real experts" that have been helping cancer patients heal for decades while running under the proverbial "radar" of conventional medicine – having been severely misdiagnosed as charlatans and quacks.

No, these "alternative" practitioners are the real "conventional" healers of our time. Taking what God gave us to repair our bodies when they break down, they have proven themselves to be the "go-to" experts when cancer strikes.

Ladies and Gentlemen, it's time to question the status quo of cancer treatment. In fact, it's far past time to challenge "business as usual." The reasoning is clear and the evidence is there – in fact, it's everywhere.

CHAPTER TWELVE

"THE FUTURE:
CANCER ON THE ROPES"

"Just as we are amused today at the primitive medical practices of history, future generations surely will look back at our own era and cringe at the senseless cutting, burning and poisoning that now passes for medical science."
G. Edward Griffin – *World Without Cancer*

PRESIDENT Richard M. Nixon officially declared the "War on Cancer" through the National Cancer Act of 1971. Forty years later, and by any logical measure, this war has been lost. It is long past time for conventional research and medicine to run the white flag up the pole and confess that virtually nothing has been accomplished and that cancer has beaten them. The trillion-dollar cancer industry should also admit that they have no new weapons or strategies to wage battle on any front regarding treatments or therapies.

Finally, this conglomeration of governmental agencies, medical associations, and international drug companies should own up to the death and destruction that they have wreaked on cancer patients and their families over the last four decades since this "pseudo crusade" began. Business as usual must stop and the status quo must change.

The American Cancer Society (ACS) was founded in 1913 as the American Society for the Control of Cancer. It was renamed the ACS in 1945. The National Cancer Institute was inaugurated in 1937. Most reading this book were not even born when these organizations opened and took root. They have grown to be colossal, multi-billion dollar, mega-businesses. The ACS is the largest, non-religious, private charity in the world with a several billion dollar annual budget and billions of dollars in assets. The sad thing is that most of this money is not utilized to help in the prevention, education or cure for cancer. Instead, the majority of its income is used to fund the massive overhead that has become common-place in the "business" of cancer. This is a matter of public record and can be verified by looking at their annual IRS Form 990 Return.

Please note, however, that although cancer has become a mega-business that has been utterly corrupted by power and greed, I am not "finger pointing" at the dedicated doctors, nurses, and other healthcare practitioners who are diligently working to create genuine healing for their patients. These will take no offense – they know who they are, and can stand proudly in the work they are doing.

No, the system is at fault. We (America – and, indeed, the rest of the World) have created a "Frankenstein" of cancer care and treatment that has turned on us. This "scarecrow" from Oz doesn't have a brain and is wallowing peacefully in the putrid ocean of perceived omnipotence and avarice. And, if it remains this way, Americans have virtually no health or healing chance and cancer will proliferate – even more so than it does today.

You've seen the statistics. Up to a million and a half of us in the United States will be diagnosed with cancer this year. Many others will, unknow-ingly, be "growing, fertilizing, and feeding" it within their bodies. More Americans will die of cancer from January to December than perished in World War II, the Korean War, and the Vietnam War – combined. A cancer victim dies of this disease every minute of every day of every week of every month of every year. The International Agency for Research on Cancer (IARC) published their "New World Cancer Report" in December of 2008 that estimates 20-26 million new cancer diagnosis and

13-17 *million* deaths by the year 2030. That is nearly *triple* the year 2000 numbers! Yeah, there's cancer prevention and control for you.

Tell me – when does this end? Or does it? When does it get so bad that we decide to do something about it? After all, as you have just witnessed through the pages of this book, we do, in fact, know what heals us and how to deal with this man-made plague.

As early as the 1930's, Royal Raymond Rife, Harry Hoxsey, Linus Pauling, Johanna Budwig, Max Gerson, Ernst Krebs, William Kelley, et al., had this "cancer thing" figured out. And they paid the price for forwarding the natural therapies, foods, nutrients, and protocols that allowed the human body to defeat this disease – and many others. These dedicated professionals, and countless more, spent their lives researching and studying the causes – and resultant "cures" – for cancer, and were rewarded by the establishment with threats, censure, discrediting, and being hounded and run out of business – and, if you can even imagine it in a "free" country – sometimes worse.

What in the world has become of us? And how, on God's green earth, have we allowed this to happen? We must, collectively, answer these questions before we can ever hope to positively affect the future of cancer and its treatments. We simply cannot go on the way we have. Albert Einstein once said that "the definition of insanity is doing the same thing over and over again and expecting different results." And yet we continue to ply cancer patients with surgery, chemotherapy, radiation and drugs – and they die. *What can we possibly be thinking?*

The "breath" of ineffective, conventional treatments for cancer must be stopped – literally, the life must be "choked" out of them. And lifeless things should be buried. In the last chapter Dr. Andrew Weil was quoted as saying that "radiation and chemotherapy are crude treatments that will be obsolete before long." In 1987, Dr. Alan Levin, Professor of Immunology at the University of California Medical School, stated,

"Most cancer patients in this country die of chemotherapy. Chemotherapy does not eliminate breast, colon or lung cancers. The fact has been documented for over a decade…Women with breast cancer are likely to die faster with chemotherapy than without it." (Source: www.starthealthylife. com website).

From the www.cancerinform.org website (and published in many, many cancer resource documents):

"In 1986, McGill Cancer Center scientists sent a questionnaire to 118 doctors who treated non-small-cell lung cancer. More than three quarters of them recruited patients and carried out trials of toxic drugs for lung cancer. They were asked to imagine that they themselves had cancer, and were asked which of six current trials they themselves would choose. Of the 79 respondents, 64 said they would not consent to be in a trial containing cisplatin, a common chemotherapy drug. Fifty-eight found all the trials unacceptable. Their reasons? The ineffectiveness of chemotherapy and its unacceptable degree of toxicity."

Friends, that's *73%* of oncologists (those who dispense chemotherapy) that said they would not undergo the *very* treatments that they recommend and administer – *no matter what!!*

How can we possibly believe, conceive, or perceive that there is any future for chemotherapy (or radiation therapy) as a treatment for cancer? What will it take to convince us?

Thomas Edison – remember him? This great American inventor was quoted as saying that "the doctor of the future will give no medicine, but will interest his patients in the care of the human frame, in diet and in the cause and prevention of disease." And that's *exactly* where the future of cancer treatment and cure lies.

Is this a secret? You would think so. Ever since Hippocrates said, "Let thy food be thy medicine," there appears to have been an ever-building conspiracy to "dumb-down" our food with unnatural and synthetic preservatives and additives and to replace its medicinal uses with ever more man-made pharmaceuticals.

The cat is out of the bag now, however. The huge and solid rock of "alternative medicine" (thy food) is rolling down the steep hill of public opinion and headed straight for the crumbling building that is conventional cancer therapy. The American public doesn't seem to be so dumb after all. They have been fooled for a time (too long) by the smoke and mirrors of allopathic medicine, its purveyors and supporters. But now, the jig is up, the beans have been spilled, and the season for slash, burn, and poison is ending.

If the human body really does have the ability to heal itself when given the proper nutrients, water, supplements and protocols (and most believe that it does), then we really need to ask ourselves the following question: Is cancer really a medical problem, or a political one? I would purport to you that it is the latter. If, indeed, the politics are extracted from this disease, the power and money become non-issues and the real remedies are revealed and accepted. And these healing mechanisms are natural, efficacious, and non-toxic. They build and restore the immune system, flush out poisons, efficiently and effectively process nutrients, and create homeostasis within the body.

So, let's do this. Let's separate the "us versus them" mentality from the anti-cancer equation and focus on what is really important, and what the title of this book suggests: killing cancer – not people. If we can wrap our minds around this concept and jettison all the remaining "falderal" – the answer to cancer will appear, even to those who don't want to see it.

So, now accepting that cancer really is on the ropes and conventional medical therapies and treatments are on their way out, I want to give you the shopping list of exactly what is on the horizon in the form of natural supplements, foods, treatments, and immunotherapies that will make a significant difference in the radically changed and prolonged lives of cancer patients.

Of course, this summary will be far from complete. There are many supplements and protocols currently available that have not been mentioned in this writing. That does not mean that they are not good or effective. It simply means that I was limited to time and space and chose what I believed (through personal use, interviews, testimonies, and research) to be the most effective and proven – and what I would use and do if I had cancer. As stated in earlier chapters, do your own research, mind your homework, question everything, then select what you believe will work best for you. What has been recommended herein has been tried and proven by tens of thousands of cancer patients – and most of them, when adhering to the protocols, have healed.

Nothing will ever improve on Mother Nature. The earth provides what we need to survive, thrive and heal. Plant extracts are the basis for most medicines. But instead of using them directly or in homeopathic solutions, man – in his arrogance – has chosen to try to synthesize these ingredients for fun and profit. Largely, it hasn't worked. Instead, we have produced drugs that have horrific side effects for which more drugs are required. Do you remember the commercial that exclaims, "It's not nice to fool Mother Nature?" Well, it's not and she's ticked.

While a few are poisonous and some not palatable, most plants on this earth are chock full of phytonutrients, vitamins, minerals, enzymes, and other valuable substances that, when used as a whole extract and not fractionated, are very effective in maintaining cellular health within the human species. Although I believe that God put animals on this earth and made them available for us to eat, we were largely meant to be vegetarians. Our digestive systems testify to this. Understanding and forwarding through this writing that the human body, with a very strong immune system, has the ability to heal itself, I submit to you that a large part of man's answer to healing cancer (and preventing it) lies within the use of these plant foods and extracts.

Even now, thousands of researchers are evaluating thousands of plants – their leaves, roots, stems, and flowers – and utilizing the individual selected extractions "in vitro" to test for anti-cancer characteristics. Unfortunately, many are in pharmaceutical labs (remember graviola) and destined to be new drugs. I am aware of several of these investigations (non-drug) and am indirectly involved in two. These two are outlined as follows:

Extract A, called the "Karkinos Extract," was actually developed from a South American plant species during the late 1950's and early 1960's. It went through significant patient testing (end stage cancer) and was shown to alleviate all the pain associated with the disease within 24-48 hours of administration. In addition, it put all patients who received it (who weren't almost dead from conventional therapies) into permanent remission. I'm not calling it a cure. But they did. Following is a brief description of the observational results:

1 – "Fast, thorough control of pain, along with a marked improve-
    ment of the general condition of the patient, that can be
    accurately described as vanishing of the symptomatic compo-
    nents of tumoral cachexia; recovery of the color of the face, of
    the appetite, of the ability to sleep, of physical energy, and of
    body weight. A noticeable but limited effect of euphoria was also
    observed.

2 – "Within 15 days from the date administration started, incip-
    ient tumor remission was observed to be taking place in all
    of the patients under treatment, regardless of type of cancer.
    The patients who had irreversible damage in vital organs did
    not survive; however, they reached the exitus letalis without

experiencing pain and in a general condition and state of mind that made them believe they were recovering. The patients who didn't have such irreversible damage, eventually recovered after several months under treatment.

3 – "At the end of the first year of clinical trials, the authorization to continue with them was cancelled. The work continued, however, at a private medical practice for a period of more than twenty years.

4 – "The response to the treatment was the same in all cases without exception, with just a few relapses that were satisfactorily resolved. The relapses were not by way of new or resuming tumoral growths, but of renewed presence of the primary causal factor, the failing of a main detoxication function, verifiable by means of specific tests in urine and blood. Many of the patients treated remained under observation for several years, with periodic administration of those tests, which had been designed for detecting the biochemical dysfunction to which prime causality was, and is – still nowadays – attributed. This extract was 'shelved' (think traditional medicine threats and pressure) for decades and is just now being reintroduced, through its proprietary formula, to new testing and verification."

There's that dang "empirical evidence" again.

Extract B, which I'll call the "AAG Extract," has not been the subject of a comprehensive investigation, as was the case of the "Karkinos Extract." Some time after an observation that animals ingesting this specific plant had their cancerous tumors resolved (sounds like Hoxsey – but is not), an extract was produced from the plant leaves and tried by direct injection in malignant growths. Within two to five days on average, the tumors would shrink, "dry-up," and subsequently fall off (external animal tumors), leaving an empty space where previously located, without further consequences. These observations and experimentation took place at a cattle ranch by a veterinarian doctor in 1988:

"Around 1995, a homeopathic solution was made from the extract to try on a few cancer patients with a terminal prognosis who had not responded to conventional treatments, including chemotherapy. Being in the countryside, the availability of sophisticated means for cancer treatment, and economic means to pay for them, even if available, were scarce – to say the least.

"The first results were positive and, as the news circulated, more people with cancer, treated and untreated, began asking for the product to treat themselves.

"Over the years since 1995, the number of patients treated may be in the neighborhood of 15,000 – or more. In many cases, the patients, once their condition was under control, went back to the physicians who had initially treated them and were notified that they were free of cancer. Or, at least, free of detectable malignant growths, which is not necessarily equal to being free of cancer. No evidence of adverse effects was ever produced."

Many thanks to Dr. Eduardo De la Maria, Ph.D., for this data produced and quoted from his research report.

Hopefully, additional testing will "prove-out" these extracts once again and they will be brought to the anti-cancer marketplace soon. Rest assured that the FDA and the pharmaceutical industry will bring all pressure to bear to keep these products from afflicted cancer patients and prosecute any and all who dare to forward these "unapproved drugs."

Much similar testing is occurring throughout the world, although not in conventionally approved clinical trials. No, the FDA backed approval committees would never stand for that. The majority of this type of research is being done in out-of-the-way places or in countries that can't be reached or bothered by the long arm of U.S. law. Since these "new medicines" are natural and non-toxic, populations that are now prone to cancer because they have begun adapting to a "Western Diet," are ideal and grateful candidates and many have healing experiences as described with the two extracts above.

Additional research (scientific – just not clinical) is currently in process here in the United States regarding known supplements and foods – and combinations thereof. We don't hear much about this because those participating are more interested in finding solutions than making money. They have personal histories or testimonies involving cancer and are seeking answers that traditional research and medicine are not providing. You won't find these people tied up in genome or gene experiments that will never give us a solution to cancer. No, these dedicated souls are doing the real work and seeking the answers (and finding them) that have, for so long, been hiding in the seemingly "alternate universe" outside of conventional existence. It doesn't take the proverbial rocket scientist to realize that you don't look for math answers in your geography book. Please, someone rush out and tell that to the National Institutes of Health.

Studies involving combinations of DMSO with several other nutrients and supplements are underway. As previously mentioned, individual blood/colostrum/transfer factor vaccines are being developed and tested in Mexico. Cuban scorpion venom is currently being used and touted as a cancer "cure" by many. There are other products and protocols being investigated that are secret and "underground" and their originators will not yet speak of them – nor can I at this point in time. I am bolstered by the fact that study and research for alternative and natural remedies for cancer continues despite the threats from our government and private industry. You go, girls – and guys.

An amazing amount of work in electromedicine is being accomplished as the quest to duplicate the previous success of Royal Raymond

Rife continues. Some call this "energy medicine" and the equipment runs the gamut from Hulda Clark's "Zappers" and the previously evaluated GB-4000, to the Vibe Machines that are designed to raise the vibrational levels of the body to the highest oscillations, where they initially functioned. These devices use a combination of ozone, argon, krypton and water vapor and, when turned on, will light incandescent bulbs 10 feet away. Even though it is kind of an eerie feeling sitting in front of one of these while operational, my experience was peaceful and rewarding. Many whom I have spoken with swear by these machines for a variety of illnesses.

Other products boast of therapeutic benefits in energy medicine, such as Enercel®, that is advertised as "a compound whose function regenerates the mitochondria, producing white blood cells that target and destroy disease" (www.enercel.org). We know that these functions boost the immune system which, in turn, benefits cancer patients.

All things considered, in the final analysis, if we are sincere about ultimately and conclusively defeating cancer, the real answer that we seek is "prevention." If we can visualize (synthetically – or not) the end of this madness, this seemingly eternal controversy over what really works – and what doesn't – for sufferers of this disease, we must pull to the surface the incontrovertible evidence that what "heals" cancer also "prevents" it, and vice versa. With this truth in our "alternative" medicine bag, cancer can – and will – become a non-issue in our lifetimes. We simply must embrace the sweetness and effectiveness of natural, non-toxic therapies and treatments. After all, what worked for our ancestors (and my Great Hekawi Grandmother) was not drugs and poison. No, they ate right, drank good water, and made full use of the plant kingdom to heal themselves when they were sick. And the inarguable fact is that your immune system will do it for you, even with cancer, if you give it the opportunity. Most importantly, now that you know this, don't forget it – and don't be "bullied" by those who, in their ignorance, say it isn't so.

I sincerely believe that the future for cancer patients lies in the tenants of this book. If I didn't believe that, if I wasn't prepared to practice what I preach, if I didn't do many of these things right now – without cancer – I wouldn't recommend them to you. Because of that and, before moving on to the final chapter, let me first summarize what I have said I would do if I were diagnosed with cancer today. Keep in mind that, almost exclusively, this would include "any" type of cancer at "any" stage.

First of all, I would not have surgery unless it was absolutely and imminently necessary to save my life (tumor blocking bile duct, arterial interference, etc). I would not undergo chemotherapy or radiation therapy under any circumstances – except targeted, insulin potentiation therapy (IPT) if it was absolutely necessary to shrink a tumor immediately to save my life (not likely).

I would stop eating all sugar, all packaged foods, all meat (in most instances) and dairy products, trans fats, hydrogenated oils, table salt, black pepper, anything refined (flours), peanuts, cashews, corn (fungus), and eggs (unless pregnant), and stop drinking tap water, alcohol, and coffee (with exceptions). I would immediately cease using fluoridated toothpaste (use non-aluminized baking soda instead) and all personal care products with chemicals that could harm me. I would embrace an alkaline diet high in raw vegetables and would juice these, as well. Wheatgrass juice and a good barley leaf supplement would be a multi-daily staple of my treat-ment. I would drink ionized water (so important for cancer patients) or, if that was not available, only quality well or spring water. I would imme-diately detox my colon, liver and gallbladder and do a parasite cleanse. I would spend at least 15 minutes to a half hour in the sun every day – but not get sunburned – and use *no* tanning lotions or burn protection.

I would do an initial "Navarro Urine Test" and, subsequently, make it an every-other-month event to chart the remission of cancer in my body. I would find an "advocate" – or ten – who would support me, without reservation, through this "cancer experience" that I intend to win. My next step would be to review the supplement list in Chapter Five, order them, and begin these protocols – especially vitamin D3 and iodine.

If unable to care for myself or administer the appropriate diet and protocols, I would seriously consider one of the Chapter Seven inpatient or outpatient clinics and would hire a cancer coach. In fact, I would hire a cancer coach, regardless of the seriousness of my condition. If I were a late Stage III or Stage IV cancer patient, I would incorporate an electro-medicine machine (GB-4000) into my treatment and undergo Ultraviolet Blood Irradiation therapy given through a qualified alternative physician. Despite the fact that I *would want* to, I *wouldn't* forget the coffee enemas. If I was still upwardly mobile and able, I would get as much exercise as was comfortable for me and would use a rebounder a couple of times a day to help drain my lymphatic system.

And, I would give myself a serious attitude adjustment, understanding that I have a plan in place – one that I know can work for me – and would have complete confidence that I would heal.

This is a brief summary of the first eleven chapters. Herein lies a protocol that has worked for tens of thousands to help them resolve their cancers. In most instances – and if followed closely (no cheating) – it works to build and enhance the immune system, which is truly our only hope of beating cancer.

Buy into it; stick with it; *heal.*

On to lucky Chapter Thirteen.

CHAPTER THIRTEEN

"THE AMERICAN ANTI-CANCER INSTITUTE, UNIVERSITY, AND IMMUNE CLINIC"

"What you are about to read will shock you. It is a story of oncologists lying to parents about the efficacy of their therapy and using coercive tactics such as threats of court orders to take children and submit them to treatments that they know are torturous and ineffective. We were told, not asked, but told that we had 30 days from Alexander's surgeries to start chemo. We were told that chemo would offer Alexander a good chance of survival. We were told that he would be getting a new chemo protocol with 'state-of-the-art' drugs. And we were warned that if we did not bring Alexander in for chemotherapy a court order would be forthcoming so that the oncologists could take him from us and administer these poisons without our approval. We were lied to and threatened so that oncologists could fill our son with deadly ineffective poisons that simply shortened his life and made his last days on earth a living hell."

No Rights For a Child Diagnosed With Cancer
Raphaele & Michael Horwin

WHILE I firmly believe that conventional medicine has lost the war on cancer, I do not maintain that "alternative medicine" can, as yet, claim victory. However, I now can conceive of the day that my children will have the freedom to select any treatments, therapies or protocols to deal with their own individual health issues.

The American people are a resilient bunch. Back us into a corner and we'll come out fighting – no matter how tough you think you are. Well folks, we have been literally "cornered" through a "sick-care" scandal (with a cancer of its own) that has blatantly squandered trillions of taxpayer dollars over the past five decades and produced virtually nothing. We have been to that mountaintop and, unlike the revered Dr. Martin Luther King, we have seen no promised land.

The "promise" of traditional cancer research has always been "the cure." And it still is today, despite the "empirical" proof that no such remedy is in sight on the allopathic radar screen. We continue, however, to eat up the cancer-cure rhetoric and the public is insidiously and perpetually sucked into the yearly announcements of major advancements in cancer research – those continuous missives that put the long elusive cure right around the corner. What they don't tell you is that the corner is somewhere on Pluto (Pluto don't get no respect). But I digress.

The fact is that what we really need to know about the successful treatment of cancer – we *already* know. The tools we require to defeat this disease are already in the toolbox. The answer to cancer no longer begs the question. So now that we "know what we know" to be true, right, efficacious, and healing, where do we go from here? How do we go forward? What's the plan of attack? Herein lies the problem.

We have already defined alternative medicine as really the misnomer for true conventional medicine. After all, what's more traditional than using natural ingredients to prevent and heal disease? And what's more "alternative" than putting poison and radiation (things we are told as children to avoid at all costs) into the body to heal cancer?

Unfortunately (referring to the problem), "as labeled" alternative medicine is beginning its long hoped for phase of exponential growth in a severely fragmented state. While more and more dedicated and serious people and businesses are involved in this field each year, many are doing their own thing, selling their proprietary products, advancing their individual equipment, treatments, supplements and therapies with little regard for the movement as a whole. While this appears to be good for business on a primary level, it transfers no momentum to the slowly moving pendulum of natural health care and prevention that needs to complete the upswing (credibility), before it can impel itself, at an ever-increasing speed, through the down-swing of acceptance and widespread implementation through its practical application.

In other words, we need to work together, support like-mindedness, and ally with one another to become a force to be reckoned with. The approach must be streamlined, the "fluff" shucked, the hucksters exposed, the fear controlled, and the truth forwarded.

Conventional medicine has now latched onto "buzz" phrases in an effort to convince Americans that they are listening and changing to incorporate alternatives into their allopathic regimens. Being bantered about now by the same medical association that brought chemo and radiation to a theater near you, are the marketing pieces featuring "Complimentary and Alternative Medicine," or CAM, and "Integrative Medicine." The idea here is that conventional treatments are now including portions of alternative medicine to "compliment" the traditional therapies and "integrating" them into allopathic cancer procedures.

While I laud our current medical convention for promoting prayer, counselors, and better diets for our inflicted brethren, don't be fooled into believing for a second that this resembles choice in medicine or true alternative treatment (with a few exceptions). To be fair, a few have gone a little further than this and have realized that a basic alkaline diet is what a cancer patient requires. And while it will help, this protocol is seriously deflected by round after round of chemotherapy and radiation treatment. Having said that, it's much better than the standard hospital fare of soda pop and sugared protein drinks. No need to go through that again. Just beware that the medical locations advertising CAM and IM are largely – if not mostly – conventional treatment facilities.

This apparent change in marketing ploys by cancer care centers and hospitals is an effort, not so much to offer alternative therapies, as it is to splinter and dilute the aspirations of those who are really trying to forward the effective protocols. If it can be perceived that local entities are offering the best of both worlds, perhaps cancer sufferers can be convinced that their chances are better within these facilities. And while, indeed, the healing opportunity might be slightly increased there, it won't be significant, as conventional treatments are still the mainstay.

Referring back to the concept that the alternative cancer community must discover a way to find common ground and bind together – enter the American Anti-Cancer Institute (AACI), the American Anti-Cancer University, and the American Anti-Cancer Immune Clinic.

The idea behind the AACI – with it's teaching and clinical subsidiaries – was born from the notion that a "clearing house" for all things cancer and anti-cancer was necessary to forge into being an alliance of those really interested in bringing an end to cancer as we know it – and actually working to make that happen.

Hence, a new IRS designated 501©(3), not-for-profit entity was formed with a mission to coordinate research of non-allopathic cancer treatments, therapies, protocols, and supplements; conduct educational and preventative cancer programs and make them available to the general public (at no cost through the University); promote alternative cancer treatments that have been proven to be efficacious for cancer patients; become the clearing house for all viable methodologies, information, and non-conventional treatments regarding cancer; and to produce and promote genuine "cures" within ten years. And in a very short period of time, most of this has already been accomplished.

The AACI is essentially an intellectual and collaborative partnership between actual cancer patients and alternative medical doctors, cancer specialists, researchers and scientists.

Experimental technologies and treatments are currently being explored and tested for their efficacy and forwarded or discarded based upon proven promise to support longevity, quality of life, and healing for cancer sufferers.

This organization is currently partnering with – and setting up grant programs to fund – companies and institutions that promote, research, test, and prove scientific methodologies to treat cancer and, ultimately, bring healing without surgery, chemotherapy, radiation or drugs. Its vision encapsulates a new cancer health "cure" system – devoid of unproven, life-ending therapies that do little to help cancer victims but much to promote a multi-trillion dollar industry that *exists to exist.* And from the www.americanaci.org website and the AACI "Vision Statement," comes the following:

"The American Anti-Cancer Institute is predicting the death of cancer as we know it, will work diligently to kill it and, will publish the death certificate to the American Public within ten years."

One would naturally think this to be a pretty outrageous statement – if one was not familiar with the facts. Now that you know the real truth surrounding cancer, its causes and prevention, you realize that this is not only very doable but, in fact, already being done.

The real hope for cancer lies in this philosophy and quest. And the AACI, in conjunction with a myriad of other institutes and foundations like the Independent Cancer Research Foundation, the American Anti-Cancer Society, the Cancer Control Society, and literally hundreds of others willing to ally against cancer and its failed convention, will see this process through to fruition in short order.

So, what's the plan? Once again, glad you asked.

The American Anti-Cancer Institute has on its drawing board a 40-50 acre "Anti-Cancer Campus" whose design has already been mostly completed. This one hundred twenty-five million dollar effort will be funded largely through a multi-faceted capital campaign that will begin in the Spring of 2011.

This campus will include the 30,000 square foot, three-story, American Anti-Cancer Institute; the 30,000 square foot, three- story, American Anti-Cancer University; and the 160,000 square foot, eight-story, American Anti-Cancer Immune Clinic. In addition, a 20,000 square foot cafeteria and public restaurant (featuring anti-cancer foods) will support the nutritional needs of the Clinic's cancer patients. Up to ten acres of certified organic gardens will supply vegetables to the kitchens and 2-3 acres of greenhouses will grow the wheatgrass and barleygrass for onsite consumption. Numerous other support buildings are planned.

Imagine, if you will, an affordable place where cancer victims can go to be treated through natural means; a safe haven where all of their needs can be met – nutritional, educational, and medical – at less than a tenth of the cost of conventional cancer treatment and care. I know, I know – it's hard to conceive and even harder to believe that allopathic concerns would even "allow" it to happen. But it will – you can count on it. How? Common Americans like you and me will fund it. Why? Because it's the right thing to do and the right time to do it.

Friends, we need to take charge of our health, cancer or not. Just like my mother "really" knew the two packs of cigarettes she was smoking daily were not good for her, we also are very aware (more so now) that what we eat, what we drink, what we breathe, and how we live, contribute to our longevity and quality of life.

Unfortunately, we are a chronically "sick" society that lives in whatever manner we please and then hopes that the doc has the magic pill when we start to fail. Well, he doesn't. Medicine has come a long way in the past 50 years, thanks largely to diagnostic equipment and drugs. Folks, this does not equate to quality of life — nor will it ever. No, how we live and how long we live, is primarily up to us, individually.

We really do know what to do — and how to do it. Hopefully, this book has reinforced that fact and persuaded you of this truth, whether cancer inhabits your body — or not. Without the proper plan — statistics say it will.

So, as the singers "Dale and Grace" once said, "I'm leaving it all up to you." Isn't this a great country! You get to do whatever you darn well please. And I'll say it again. Choose wisely my Friends.

And, finally, the answer is "yes." The "Hekawis" *were* the Indian Tribe from the television series and book "F Troop." And that's the only "non-truth" in this book. Sorry Gram.

EPILOGUE

"Kites rise highest against the wind – not with it."

Sir Winston Churchill

N O one has the right to tell you what to do – especially if you have cancer. That's a decision you must make for and by yourself.

While I would never accuse someone of taking or making that life-changing resolution lightly, I know for a fact that most of us **do not** have all the pertinent and correct information to make it accurately or correctly. How do I know that? Simply because most people, due to their lack of understanding concerning the facts surrounding cancer and how it is really healed, make the **wrong** decision. And although it's not their fault, for many of these, the statistics **prove** that it will cost them their lives.

This deeply saddens me and there are those who asked me not to say it this way. "People will be angry, they will be offended by these accusations and the way you present them," they said. My response was that they didn't give the American people enough credit. Although the truth sometimes hurts and we wish it could be different, we still want to know it and are better off when we do.

Where have we heard "and the truth shall set you free?" When did that cease to be the mantra of a society that was built on both truth and individual freedom? No, I think that deep down people want candor, unvarnished veritableness, the straight poop. They are tired of being deceived, weary of impropriety, sick of the "business as usual" mentality that pervades our government entities and our unchallenged and competition-free "sick-care" system.

In the pages that you have just read, this candor and truth is exactly what you have gotten – in a plan and protocol that I would follow if I had cancer; the real gospel about what works and what doesn't; whether you like it or not. I understand that there are some who won't like it; no, they won't care for it at all.

There are those who will believe that I have "dissed" traditional and conventional medicine. They would be half right – but they are probably more than half mad. Unquestionably, I have maligned a *system* that is not working and has no functional capacity to do so for chronically ill cancer patients. The proof of the failure that is American "health care" today has been presented in this work and is additionally produced in volumes of white papers, clinical research, news reports, and our overall dismal world ranking of 37th by the World Health Organization (WHO) – in their year 2000 report, *Health Systems: Improving Performance* – just above Slovenia and right below Costa Rica.

Proof here comes from the January 6th, 2010 edition of the *New England Journal of Medicine* – and is forwarded by *medical doctors* as follows:

"Despite the claim by many in the U.S. health policy community that the international comparison is not useful because of the uniqueness of the United States, the rankings have figured prominently in many arenas. It is hard to ignore that in 2006, the United States was number 1 in terms of health care spending per capita but ranked 39th for infant mortality, 43rd for adult female mortality, 42nd for adult male mortality, and 36th for life expectancy. These facts have fueled a question now being discussed in academic circles, as well as by government and the public: Why do we spend so much to get so little?"

Why indeed?

While it could be said that I have maligned a traditional and conventional medical **system** that has not served the American Public well, what I have **certainly not** done herein, nor would I, is to intentionally slander our dedicated health care workers – the doctors, nurses, technicians, administrators, etc. – specifically, those who labor every day with heavy hearts in an attempt to bring healing to those who suffer immeasurably from cancer and its standard treatments. No, I blame the system that allows cancer to happen, to proliferate, to maim and to kill. It just shouldn't be so. In that sense, the sense that, willingly or unknowingly we all play some part in this arrangement, we are inarguably all to blame. Hopefully, this writing will be the beginning of an awareness of what works and what doesn't; what is proven and what isn't.

People know the difference between right and wrong – no matter which they follow. Throughout our lives, we are constantly and consistently taught to do what is right. Although there are occasions that we may vary from that pathway, most of us generally seek to be redirected onto the road through life that is truth and righteousness. This is not an attempt to wax philosophically. Rather, it is a plea to do this same thing when caring for your own health and well being when faced with the scourge of cancer.

Seek what is right. Search for what is proven. Go in quest of the real healing mechanisms for cancer. Refuse to settle for less. Don't buckle under to the status quo or to the "brow beating" of someone who has absolutely nothing at stake. No, choose life, then fight like heck for it.

I believe you made a major investment when you bought this book. And I don't just mean the dollars you spent, but rather the endowment that is being produced and paying dividends through the knowledge and understanding that there is a better and more effective way to treat cancer. This is an investment whose yield is exponential. Please, pay it forward.

As you do, keep in mind that there is an ever-growing presence of those so-called "alternative" practitioners and researchers that have resolved to make the real difference in this war on cancer. And they need help. As previously mentioned, they will not get it from any source connected in any way to conventional research or medicine. There will be no grants forthcoming from traditional institutions or foundations, and certainly not from governmental agencies. No, their diligence and work goes unrecognized, unrewarded, and unfunded. They are the "Rodney Dangerfields" of cancer care and cure. They just don't get no respect.

I'm asking you to not only respect them – but to help them, as well. For without you, sans the average "Joe," the common man and woman in America and throughout the world, these purveyors of the truth about cancer and its healing realities will go the way of the blacksmith.

Please consider becoming a volunteer if you have the time or are persuaded by the righteousness of this movement. I sincerely hope that you are. Find an organization that is championing the true tenants encompassing cancer and give them some of your time.

Of equal importance, and you knew this was coming, reach into your pocket (by way of your heart) and give a few bucks to these struggling organizations, researchers, and institutions that are making the *"real"* difference for cancer patients. Small, individual donations are often the only way they stay afloat. Do a little of your own research and choose who you would like to help.

The American Anti-Cancer Institute was recognized and "defined" in Chapter 13. This organization is worthy of your support. For as little as one dollar per month you could become a member of the "Curative Power of One" which recognizes that "one" person, giving "one" dollar, results in thousands of people giving tens of thousands of dollars (powers of one) that sustains the research that heals cancer patients.

Another call to action is the *One Million Enemies of Cancer*, a world-wide collection of those of us who are willing to pony-up a couple of dollars a month – every month – to change the face of cancer care as we know it. Imagine, if you will, one million (or more) enemies of cancer, giving only $5 per month, generating $5 million each and every month that would, inevitably, make these "alternative medicine" treatments, therapies, and protocols available to all who seek them. Tell me, who can't give this *small* amount to make this *huge* difference?

I hope you "are in." I am. All of the net proceeds from the sale of this book will go to the American Anti-Cancer Institute. I figured if I was going to "talk the talk," I'd better "walk the walk."

Please go to the web address below to become an integral part of the real and true "answer to cancer" and a partner with the AACI through the *Curative Power of One* and/or the *One Million Enemies of Cancer*.

www.americanaci.org/articlepage.aspx?categoryID=9

If you see any politics or conspiracy theory in all of this, please look past them, as they are unintended.

This book is solely meant to help cancer patients and forward the truth about this disease and the methods with which to heal it. There are no ulterior motives hidden or implied.

Thank you for purchasing this work and please accept my sincere appreciation for your continued support of anti-cancer research and the real solutions for cancer patients.

It is with much sadness that I report the death of the infant child whose story I told at the beginning of Chapter Seven – after a very short 5 and one half months of life. My deepest sympathy to his family.

Bob Wright

EPILOGUE TWO

NEW ON THE HORIZON:
ALTERNATIVE TREATMENT FOR PEDIATRIC CANCER? HOW TO AVOID EVERY PARENT'S WORST NIGHTMARE

"RUN FOR THE BORDER"

"If children have the ability to ignore all odds and percentages, then maybe we can all learn from them. When you think about it, what other choice is there but to hope? We have two options, medically and emotionally: give up or fight like hell."

Lance Armstrong

This book would not be complete without including the recent tragedy related to me by Maureen Long, the founder and administrator of Camelot Cancer Care. Her clinic had just lost a six-year old patient as this book was going to press.

The names have been changed and some intimate details omitted to protect the privacy of the grieving parents. At this writing, the little boy (we will call him Howie – for Howard) had expired in his mother's arms not 48 hours before. Her grief was so raw and fresh that she was heavily sedated, possibly on suicide watch. So, we rely on recollections, para-phrased from her spoken words from the days leading up to her little son's tragic and avoidable death – as follows:

When little Howie was first diagnosed with Non-Hodgkin's Lymphoma, his parents did their research. Their first choice was alternative treatment, after they determined that the prognosis was grim and that orthodox oncology's recommended "standard of care" (toxic chemo, plus whole body radiation as prep for a bone marrow transplant) carries a horrendously high failure rate. Most patients who are coerced into submitting to this treatment succumb to either disease progression or opportunistic infections in its aftermath, because the radiation destroys the immune system – and then the immune suppressant drugs prevent the rebuilding of it – paving the way for progression of the cancer.

In short, it is a recipe for failure and disaster that should be rejected by anyone on grounds of simple logic and reasoning. Yet, this standard of care is defended and continues to be practiced by mainstream oncology, despite the fact that the long-term survival rate following this procedure is vanishingly small.

But, let's get back to the story. When Howie's parents expressed their desire to seek out alternative treatment, they were told that children do not have the same treatment choice options as adults and, unless they submitted their child to the procedure recommended by the oncologist, social services would take action. Translation: a court order seizing custody and placing the child in foster care to ensure compliance would be issued.

At this point, the reader will be spared the heartbreaking and horrific details of how little Howie suffered from radiation poisoning; the unrelenting misery of nausea – from which there is no relief. And, of course, this injustice is compounded by the fact that the parents have no recourse for justice in a clear case of child murder (albeit, second degree, unintentional, technically – manslaughter), when the perpetrator is the state. Nothing will bring their son back and they cannot sue for the loss because (1) the "Standard of Care" has never been successfully challenged in the courts and, (2) the state can do whatever it wants to its minor children, even usurping parental rights and enforcing a standard which forecloses all hope for survival – because it is shielded by the doctrine of Sovereign Immunity.

To continue this sad story, one of the last things Howie's mother said to the Camelot Care team – the day before he died – was that she now wished she had lied to authorities, agreeing in principle to the massive whole body irradiation "as soon as we return from his Make-A-Wish trip" – and then taken him straight to Magdalena Clinic in Cancun, Mexico!

Magdalena, mentioned earlier in this book, is a satellite spin-off of Camelot Cancer Care, and is evolving into a "safe haven" for pediatric cancer patients whose parents seek to protect them from the draconian cruelty that little Howie and his helpless parents were forced to suffer. The Cancun oncologists at Magdalena are using natural, gentle, but highly potent and effective treatments similar to the Camelot therapy – and much, much more. They favor the opposite approach from mainstream oncology – boosting the immune system instead of destroying it.

Parents, please pay close attention to this. Magdalena is much better equipped to offer state-of-the-art, cutting-edge quality of care that meets the standards of ACAM (the American College of Advancement in Medicine). The location, Cancun, is in a very safe area near many affordable, all-inclusive, tropical paradise resorts – a far cry from many (but not all) border clinics. Best of all, they are outside of U.S. (FDA, AMA) jurisdiction (how sad to have to say that), with no risk of any extradition consequences trumping parental rights – because the Mexican Constitutional clause, protecting natural healing, trumps the NAFTA Treaty!

Moreover, the Mexican State of Quintana Roo (which encompasses Cozumel, Playa del Carmen and Cancun – major resort areas), in an effort to encourage medical tourism, has welcomed Magdalena and assured the protection of its patients.

If I had a child or grandchild diagnosed with cancer, I just might follow the strategy proposed by little Howie's heartbroken mother. I would definitely consider getting passports for the small patient and parents, claim to be taking a family vacation ala "Make a Wish," then vanish to the safety of the Mayan Riviera until my child was healed – or had at least received his best chance to survive. If an innocent young life is at risk, my philosophy would be that I would rather be sorry for something I did than for something I didn't do – but, in grief-stricken hindsight, should have done. And, having seen everything that I have seen involving children and cancer – I know it would, without question, be the right choice.

More was said by Howie's mother (not me, Howie's mother) that bears repeating – as a warning to other parents. But, here we have to choose our words very carefully. Many ignorant, well-meaning, mainstream oncologists encourage parents to take their children with cancer to a well-known pediatric specialty hospital named after a saint (legal counsel informs, herein, that this is the most I can safely say by way of identification and, fortunately, many hospitals are named after saints, but any reader who watches television will be able to figure it out).

Howie's parents were wise enough to decline – due to their belief that our infamous "bastion of orthodox oncology" is little more than a grist mill of death, consuming countless young lives to feed the coffers of the cancer cartel.

Harsh accusation? One need only examine the numbers of children processed into such facilities – compared to the pitifully small number of survivors who make it out, or who remain in remission 5 years later. It becomes painstakingly clear that – in this instance – the shoe fits perfectly.

So, what do I believe is the solution? The brilliant medical mavericks at Magdalena have leveled the playing field – expanding it into a safe treatment haven where children with cancer and their parents can escape the threat of having custody confiscated by the state and receive the care that truly makes a difference in surviving cancer.

Unfortunately, many parents of pediatric cancer patients are impoverished by medical expenses and the ordeal imposed upon them by the mainstream medical industry. If you know someone who has a child with cancer, please loan them this book – then refer them to the following website which can, in turn, put them in contact with patient intake coordinators for Magdalena Clinic in Cancun: www.camelotcancercare.com. Or have them call (918) 493-1011 and, if unable to get through, leave a voicemail message.

Cancun is only an hour and a half flight from the Southern United States. Flights depart daily from Los Angeles, Houston, Atlanta, and Miami.

Anyone wishing to contribute to funding the travel and treatment costs to send a child to Magdalena Clinica de Cancer, may do so by contacting the American Anti-Cancer Institute at the following email address or phone number: info@americanaci.org; 509-860-1911.

The AACI is a registered 501©(3), not-for-profit organization. All contributions are a charitable deduction, on equal par with another well-known children's cancer foundation which, although having grown into a huge, commendable organization, is in no way comparable. The difference, of course, is that AACI-sponsored kids get alternative treatment – as well as a vacation trip – and a chance to return home free of cancer.

You may ask if the foregoing is out of line or a shameless promotion – or both. You have a right to ask that. But, as I told you from the start of this journey, I will always tell you the truth – and let you know exactly what I would do. And, again, that is precisely what this story and this recommendation are about. I simply can do it no other way – there is far too much at stake when we are talking about the lives of our children. You need – and deserve – to know the facts and the truth. That's exactly what you have received here.

If you (parents) can find another clinic that successfully treats pediatric cancer – and can prove it – I say go for it. I am very sure there are others out there. Do your homework and don't just "settle" for something less than the best. When it comes to cancer, there is no second place.

I have no interest, financial or otherwise, in Camelot Cancer Care or any other clinic, retreat, hospital, or cancer care facility.

THE AUTHOR'S PERSONAL
WELLNESS PLAN

(The "No Insurance – Insurance")

LET me tell you about my individual health plan – a program that I truly believe is the best that can be found anywhere. My personal physician is Dr. Bruce West. His office is in Monterey, California. I live in the state of Washington.

I pay Dr. West $39 per year (yes, I said per YEAR) for the absolute best medical advice available – period. For my $3.25 per month, I receive his monthly newsletter that is packed with the information that really and truly serves America's sickly population, and those of us who are well and planning to stay that way. And as a subscriber, I have personal access to the good Doc via letter or fax.

From cancer to heart disease, diabetes to arthritis, vaccinations to the Mediterranean Diet, Dr. West covers the gigantic spectrum of diseases and sicknesses that penetrate our lives. And the best part is that he actually tells us what to do about it – meaning, simply, forwarding the protocols that really work to allow our bodies to heal themselves.

Although Dr. West and I have communicated many times over the past 12 years or so, we have never met. Yet, I trust him and his healing and wellness advice with no reservations. By following his general protocols (and similar programs prior to finding him), I have not been ill in over 23 years. Many would say that it is not possible to avoid all colds, flu, etc., over that extended period of time. I can tell you that it is, in fact, possible, if you do the right things.

Whether it's about prevention or a need for healing, I strenuously suggest that you find a doctor, program, or protocol that really works for *you*. Don't settle for someone or something that has absolutely no stake in whether you are sick or well, living or dying. No, instead, put your money and your faith in the products, programs, food and water that are synergistic with the human immune system and will keep you well – and heal you when you are not. Do this especially if you have cancer – or don't want to get it. I guess that would be all of us.

I don't need to remind anybody about the cost of health insurance or, as it should be called, sick insurance. The price seems to go up every other month. Nor do I need to expound on the fact that it rarely covers everything or that many cancer families are bankrupt after the stricken family member has passed.

At $39.00 per year, I can afford to buy organic foods and invest in any of the supplements mentioned in this book that help to make up the nutritional difference when my diet isn't sufficient – or if I should contract cancer. And, yes, I do have a rather expensive water ionizer (made by the Enagic® Company) on my kitchen counter – affordable only because my true "health care" costs are so low and I have no "sick care" expenses. And I thank God for that machine and the gallon of Kangen™ Water I drink daily that, I am convinced, plays *the* major role in my wellness.

Some will say that my plan is not realistic. Looking through the eyes of our country's "sick care" system, they would be right. But I would respond that I have proven that it is *very realistic*. Some will say that it may be fine for me, but not for them. Once again, I say that's bunk. If you want to be well, if you want to stay well, if you want to prevent cancer from ravaging your body – do *what is right, not what is convenient!* And the naysayers scream, once again, that it's easy for me to say. And they're right. Along side literally hundreds of thousands of other Americans, I've proven that it works – not just in theory but, in fact.

It would be irresponsible of me to tell you to cancel your health insurance (sick insurance). Do, however, research what it takes to be and stay healthy. In the final analysis, it's much less expensive than "sick care" – and you just might live a whole lot longer with a much better quality of life. And cancer hates – and avoids – healthy people.

Three dollars and twenty-five cents a month. Think about it.

Bob Wright

YOUR ATTENTION PLEASE

PLEASE consider supporting the organizations that are making a real difference through forwarding the truth about cancer, its treatments and protocols – and, with very limited funding (non-governmental), producing the unbiased research that shows what works – and what doesn't – for cancer.

The following represents the "short list." There are many more – choose who you like, but please consider these:

Great work is being done at the Cancer Control Society in Los Angeles. Meet President Frank Cousineau and co-founder Lorraine Rosenthal at the 39th Annual Convention in Universal City during the Labor Day Weekend (and every Labor Day Weekend after that). They offer great "in-kind" incentives for donations. Find them at www.cancercontrolsociety.com.

The Independent Cancer Research Foundation is doing the true cancer research that the government won't do. Each year their results are astounding and new protocols are "proven" for the fight against cancer. They are worthy of your support and are found at www.new-cancer-treatments.org.

Breast Cancer Action of San Francisco really "gets it" when it comes to education, prevention, and appropriate treatments for breast cancer. BCA vows to always make the truth available to the public – no matter what it takes. They are one of the very few organizations willing to do the work that makes a real and true difference in the lives and breast health of women. Their Web address is www.bcaction.org.

Look around, do your homework, ask the tough questions, then – as BCA states – "Think before you pink!"

CANCER QUOTES

(REMEMBER THESE)

"Cancer is a word, not a sentence."

John Diamond

"Never, never, never give up."

Winston Churchill

"One must not forget that recovery is brought about not by the physician, but by the sick man himself. He heals himself by his own power, exactly as he walks by means of his own power, or eats, or thinks, breathes or sleeps."

Georg Groddeck, 1923

...and, on the lighter side –

"I got the bill for my surgery. Now I know what those doctors were wearing masks for."

James H. Boren

"A hospital should also have a recovery room adjoining the cashier's office."

Francis O'Walsh

GLOSSARY

AACI – American Anti-Cancer Institute

ACS – American Cancer Society

Adjuvant – agent that stimulates the immune system and increases response or modifies the effect of other agents

Aflatoxin – toxic mycotoxins (from fungus) that are among the most carcinogenic substances known

Aloe Arborescens – tree-like shrub belonging to the aloe genus, used to treat cancer

Allopathic – mainstream medicine

Alternative Medicine – practice of medicine without drugs, chemicals, or radiation, using natural products and treatments

Amygdalin – vitamin B-17 in its natural form, derived from apricot kernels and other seeds; used to treat cancer

AMA – American Medical Association

Artemesinin – extract from the wormwood plant

ATP – adenosine triphosphate; a high-energy molecule that stores the energy humans need to function

Big Pharma – the pharmaceutical or drug industry

Biostatistician – statisticians that work in health-related fields

Budwig Protocol – a mixture of organic cottage cheese and organic flax oil

Cachexia – wasting syndrome, loss of weight, muscle atrophy, fatigue, weakness; often associated with the final stage of cancer

Carcinogen – cancer causing substance

Carcinoma – cancer that begins in the skin or in tissues that line or cover body organs; examples are breast, colon, liver, lung, prostate, and stomach cancer

Chelation Therapy – administration of natural substances to remove heavy metals from the body

Chemotherapy – treatment of cancer through chemicals

Chronic Disease – a disease that is long lasting or recurrent

Citric Acid Cycle – process of chemical conversion of carbohydrates, fats, and proteins to generate energy in cells

Colloidal – a mixture in which one substance is dispersed evenly within another

Colonoscopy – endoscopic examination of the colon

Colostrum – nutritious "first milk" from mother after birth; contains nutrients that establish the newborn's immune system

Conventional Medicine – the practice of medicine through surgical, radiological, and drug intervention

CT Scan – computed tomography; two-dimensional X-ray imaging

Cytotoxic – toxic or poison to cells

Debulking – surgical removal of part of a malignant tumor which cannot be completely excised

Digital Infrared Imaging – a type of infrared imaging that detects and maps radiation (heat) in the body

Distilled Water – boiled or steam condensed water that has most of the impurities and minerals removed

Ductal Carcinoma In-Situ – non-invasive breast cancer in the milk duct of the breast

Efficacy – the capacity to produce an effect – usually positive

Electrolysis – a method of using an electrical current to produce a chemical reaction

Electromedicine – science of protocols utilizing electrical current and radio waves (frequency) to kill pathogens

Empirical Evidence – objective evidence that can be replicated as opposed to theory or conjecture

Enema – procedure of injecting liquids into the rectum and colon via the anus

Energy Medicine – science of rebalancing the body's energy field through electrical and electromagnetic therapy

Epidemiologist – one who studies the frequency and distribution of diseases

Exitus Letalis – death

Extracorporeal Loop – a long venous graft that creates a loop to a recipient vessel

Falderal – a showy but worthless trifle

FDA – Food and Drug Administration

Fermentation – rotting, deriving energy anaerobically (without oxygen)

Fractionated – to divide or separate into parts

Herxheimer Reaction – a "healing crisis" when large quantities of toxins are released into the body for disposal

High Fructose Corn Syrup – cheap sugar substitute, related to obesity and insulin resistance

Hippocrates – known as the father of medicine

Holistic – health concept encapsulating all of the aspects of human health

Homeopathy – science of treating patients with natural substances that are formulated based upon individual symptoms

Homeostasis – the body's ability to regulate its inner environment

Hunzakuts – the Hunza people from Northern Pakistan

Hydrogenated Oils – saturated fatty acids

Iatrogenics – disease, illness, or death caused by medical examination or treatment

Immunotherapy – treatment of disease by enhancing immune response

Infantile Fibrosarcoma – rapidly growing malignant tumor arising from fibroblast cells during the first year of life

Insulin Potentiation Therapy – use of insulin and low dose chemotherapy to target malignant tumors

Interstitial Cystitis – chronic inflammation of the bladder wall

Ionized Water – alkaline water that is rich in hydroxyl ions and produced through electrolysis

Kreb's Cycle – process of chemical conversion of carbohydrates, fats, and proteins to generate energy in the cells (see citric acid cycle)

Lactic Acid – product of fermentation during normal metabolism, exercise, and cancer cell metabolism

Laetrile – glycoside from apricot kernels and other seeds used to treat cancer

Linseed Oil – flax oil

Logarithmic – each number value (1-10) is 10 times the magnitude of the previous number

Malignancy – cancerous tumor

Melanoma – most dangerous type of skin cancer

Metastatic – the spread of cancer

Microclusters – aggregates of water molecules

Mitochondria – powerhouse of the cell where chemical reactions and cell respiration occur

MMS – Miracle Mineral Supplement consisting of sodium chlorite mixed with a citric acid activator to make chlorine dioxide

MRI – magnetic resonance imaging; details contrast between soft tissues using magnet technology

Natural Killer Cell – immune system lymphocytes that fight infections and cancer cells

Neoplasm – tumor

NIH – National Institutes of Health

Non-Hodgkin's Lymphoma – all lymphomas (blood cancers) except Hodgkin's

Non-Small-Cell Lung Cancer – lung cancer arising from the bronchi

Omega Three Fats – unsaturated fatty acids considered essential for human health (the good fats)

Oncology – branch of medicine that deals with cancer

Organic – foods that are produced with the use of no synthetic materials or chemicals

Ozone Therapy – therapeutic use of ozone through various administrations

Pangamic Acid – vitamin B-15, also known as "instant oxygen", from apricot kernels, seeds, and other foods

Pathogen – an infectious agent; germ

PET Scan – positron emission tomography producing a three-dimensional image

pH – measure of the acidity or alkalinity of a solution or substance

Photoluminescence – treatment of the blood with various wavelengths of ultraviolet light to kill pathogens and stimulate the immune system (see ultraviolet blood irradiation – UVBI)

Phytonutrients – organic chemical compounds that occur in plants

Placebo – a simulated medical substance that can produce a controlled or measured deception

Pleomorphic – the ability of pathogens to change from one form to another, i.e., bacteria to virus, fungus to bacteria, etc.

Poly MVA – dietary supplement blend of palladium, alpha-lipoic acid, vitamins B-1, B-2, B-12, amino acids, formyl-methionine, acetyl cysteine, molybdenum, rhodium, and ruthenium

Precursor – a compound that participates in the chemical reaction that produces another compound

Probiotic – small live organisms that help maintain the microflora of the intestines

Proteolytic Enzymes – proteases that help digest proteins in food; produced in the pancreas (pancreatic enzymes)

Protomorphogens – proteins that are the fundamental building blocks of life

Radiation Treatment – treatment of cancer through the use of ionizing radiation

Reverse Osmosis – the practice of purifying water by moving it through membrane filters using pressure

Sarcoma – cancer of connective tissue cells, bones, cartilage, and fat cells

Scleroderma – connective tissue disease

Sigmoid Colon – part of the large intestine closest to the rectum and anus

Stage III Cancer – cancer that is locally advanced

Stage IV Cancer – most advanced stage of cancer; metastasized, spread to other areas of the body

Synergistic – having the ability to work together

Synthetic – prepared or made artificially; contrived

T-Cell Lymphoma – cancer of "T" cells (lymphoid system)

The Big C – cancer

The Big Three – surgery, chemotherapy, radiation

Thermography – infrared imaging that detects and maps radiation (heat) in the body

Thio-ethers – toxic products of infected root canals

Tocopherols – organic chemical compounds with vitamin E activity

Transdermally – through the skin

Trans Fats – the "bad" unsaturated fats that raise LDL cholesterol levels

Transfer Factors – tiny immune building molecules found in colostrums (first mother's milk after birth)

Ultraviolet Blood Irradiation – the treatment of blood with various wavelengths of ultraviolet light to kill pathogens and stimulate the immune system

INDEX